Plant Cytology and Genetics

NIPA® GENX ELECTRONIC RESOURCES & SOLUTIONS P. LTD.
New Delhi-110 034

About Authors

Dr. Vijay Sharma is working as Assistant Professor in Department of Genetics and Plant Breeding, Banda University of Agriculture and Technology, Banda. He did his Ph.D from Maharana Pratap University of Agriculture and Technology, Udaipur, (Rajasthan). He has experience in breeding of pulses, wheat and sesame. He has published about 15 Research Papers, 01 Book chapter, 01 Review Paper, 15 Popular articles in various journals of repute.

Dr. Kamaluddin is working as Associate Professor in Department of Genetics and Plant Breeding, Banda University of Agriculture and Technology, Banda. He did his Ph.D from Institute of Agricultural Sciences, BHU, Varanasi. He has more than 12 years' experience in teaching and research. He has about 70 publications in various journals of national and international repute, seminars and conferences. He has edited a book entitled "Plant Biotechnology: Principles and Applications" in Springer Nature Publication.

Dr. Vivek Kumar Singh is working as Senior Research Fellow in Department of Genetics and Plant Breeding, CCS Haryana Agricultural University, Hisar, He holds Ph.D. in the area of Genetics and Plant Breeding from CCS HAU, Hisar, (Haryana). He has experience in conventional breeding as well as molecular breeding of major field crops. He has published about 18 research papers, a review article, a book chapter, and various popular articles in different national and international reputed journals.

Plant Cytology and Genetics

Vijay Sharma
Assistant Professor
Department of Genetics and Plant Breeding
Banda University of Agriculture and Technology
Banda, Uttar Pradesh

Kamaluddin
Associate Professor
Department of Genetics and Plant Breeding
Banda University of Agriculture and Technology
Banda, Uttar Pradesh

Vivek Kumar Singh
Senior Research Fellow
Department of Genetics and Plant Breeding
CCS Haryana Agricultural University
Hisar, Haryana

NIPA® GENX ELECTRONIC RESOURCES & SOLUTIONS P. LTD.
New Delhi-110 034

NIPA® GENX ELECTRONIC RESOURCES & SOLUTIONS P. LTD.

101,103, Vikas Surya Plaza, CU Block
L.S.C. Market, Pitam Pura, New Delhi-110 034
Ph : +91 11 27341616, 27341717, 27341718
E-mail: newindiapublishingagency@gmail.com
web: www.nipabooks.com

For customer assistance, please contact
Phone: + 91-11-27 34 17 17
Fax: + 91-11- 27 34 16 16
E-Mail: feedbacks@nipabooks.com

ISBN: 978-81-19254-24-8

Composed and Designed by NIPA®.

Preface

Cell is the fundamental unit of life of all living organisms present on the earth. Robert Hook gave the term "Cell" while studying on cork. After discovery of the cell, interest among scientist has developed to understand the structure of the different components present in it and function of the cell. Various chemicals for staining of the cell and its components and techniques were discovered by the Cytologist during seventeenth and nineteenth century to identify chromosomes and to determine the stages of mitosis and meiosis and the life cycles of living organisms. Cytogenetics is science which deals with the study of cell particular chromosome and the function of chromosome in transmitting traits from parents to offspring. Chromosome is the physical carrier of gene which control the development of all living organism. The two key mechanism of cell division i.e. mitosis which is responsible for production of identical cells, and the meiosis is important for reproduction and heredity. Techniques have been developed, upgraded and reformed to examine chromosome of different organisms. Similarly, upgradation in microscope have allowed us to develop better understanding about the structure and function of the chromosome.

The present work is an attempt to give an understanding of the basic concepts and practical approach of the Cytology and Genetics. It covers all the spheres regarding cytology and genetics like information on microscope, cell division, Mendelian principle of heredity, linkage and their detection, gene mapping through recombination, multiple alleles, gene interaction and probability. The practical outlined in this book will benefit the students and teachers of Biological and Agricultural Sciences.

Vijay Sharma
Kamaluddin
Vivek Kumar Singh

Contents

Glossary

Albinism: Albinism means lack of pigment. It is characterised by absence of partial or complete chlorophyll in green plant.

Allele: Alternate form of a gene present on same locus on the homologous chromosome. Term allele coined by Bateson.

Alloploid: A condition in which an organism have two or more distinct genomes is termed as allopolyploidy and such organism is known as alloploid or allopolyploid. These are usually produced by chromosome doubling of interspecific hybrid.

Allosome: The chromosomes that are differ from an autosome in form, size or behaviour is known as allosome. Allosomes are also referred to as sex chromosome.

Anaphase: The stage of cell division following metaphase in which homologues chromosome or sister chromatids begin to move from equatorial plate towards the opposite poles. It is the shortest stage of mitosis.

Aneuploid: An organism or a cell having one or few chromosomes more or less than the normal disomic of the species (not a multiple of the basic number, x).

Antibody: A protein molecules that interacts specifically with an antigen molecule usually produced by a vertebrate in response to antigen.

Antigen: A proteinous substance which react with an antibody; usually it induces specific antibody production when introduced into a living vertebrate, in which not occurs naturally.

Antimutator gene: Genes which decrease the frequency of natural mutation of other genes in the same genome. Such genes are found in bacteria and bacteriophage.

Autoploid: A condition in which an organism have two or more copy of a single genome is termed as autopolyploidy and such organism is known as autoploid or autopolyploid.

Autosome: Chromosome other than sex chromosome; their kind and number is same in male and female of a species.

Back cross: The crossing of F_1 progeny to one of their parents is known as back cross.

Bivalent: The structure formed by pairing of two homologues chromosomes during pachytene onward till the beginning of anaphase I.

Cell: The basic membrane bound unit consist of all the fundamental molecules of life in all living organism. It is the basic building blocks of all living organism.

Central dogma: The formation of mRNA from DNA and then synthesis of protein from it is known as central dogma. The unidirectional flow of information in biological systems is as follows:

$$DNA \longrightarrow RNA \longrightarrow Protein.$$

Centriole: Centriole is animal cell organelle. It is cylindrical structure always present in pair; not found in plant cells. It involves in the organization of spindle fibres. .

Centromere: The localised region of chromosome where spindle fibres attach; involve in chromosome movement during cell division.

Chiasmata: The contact point of homologues chromosome between non-sister chromatids during and after diplotene, generated as a result of crossing over.

Chimera: An organism that has tissues of different genotype or origin; as a result of gene mutation, natural and artificial fusion of distinct zygotes.

Chi-square: A test of statistical significance which is used to test the significance difference between observed and expected frequencies or ratios.

Chromatid: One of two identical longitudinal produced by chromosome replication and joined at the centromere.

Chromosome: Nucleoprotein bodies composed of 300Å chromatin fibres, clearly observed during cell division, dark staining with basic dye; physical carrier of genes and genetic materials. Term chromosome was first suggested in 1888 by Waldeyer.

Cis-phase linkage: Arrangement of both the dominant alleles or recessive alleles for two traits are on the same chromosome is known as cis-phase.

Cistron: It is the largest element within a gene which is the unit of function.

Co-dominance: Both the alleles of a gene equally express themselves in the heterozygotes.

Codon: A group of three adjacent nucleotides of mRNA which codes for one amino acid.

Coincidence: It is inverse measure of interference. It is measured as a ratio between actual number of double cross overs and the expected number of double cross overs.

Colchicine: An alkaloid derived from the *Autumn crocus*; it prevent the organisation of spindle apparatus and thereby induce chromosome doubling.

Complete linkage: Linkage between genes that are so close together on a chromosome with no crossing over between them, are always inherited as a single unit, show relationship referred to as complete linkage.

Complementary gene action: Two dominant non-allelic genes capable of producing a character only when both of them are present together in the dominant state.

Crossing over: The exchange of precisely homologous segments between non-sister chromatids of homologous chromosomes that results in recombinant chromosome. It takes place during pachytene sub-stage of prophase I.

Cross pollination: The transfer of pollen grains from anther to stigma of flowers born on different plants.

Cytogenetics: A branch of biology devoted to the study of chromosome and their implications in genetics.

Cytokinesis: The division of cytoplasm into two or more parts; usually follows karyokinesis or nuclear division.

Cytoplasm: The entire content a cell outside the nucleus and enclosed within the cell membrane.

Cytoplasmic inheritance: Inheritance of characters due to the genes located in the cytoplasm e.g., mitochondria and plastids. These genes known as cytogene or plasma gene. Cytoplasmic inheritance is also known as extra-nuclear or extra-chromosomal inheritance.

Deletion: The loss of a segment from a chromosome.

Dihybrid cross: A cross is made between two true-breeding parents differing in two pairs of genes, producing an F_1 generation.

Diploid: Individual consisting two copies of chromosome complement (homologous chromosome). It is represented by 2n.

DNA: Deoxyribonucleic acid; the genetic material; serves as the template for DNA replication.

Dominant allele: In the heterozygote, one allele expresses itself at the expense of the other.

Double crossing over: It refers to the formation of two chiasmata between non-sister chromatids of homologous chromosomes. It involves three linked genes (Three point test cross).

Duplicate gene effect: Two dominant genes produce the same phenotypic effect whether they are alone or together, the alternative phenotype being produced only when both in the recessive state.

Duplication: The occurrence of a chromosome segment more than one on the same chromosome or in a genome.

Epistasis: The phenotypic expression of one gene is masked by another non-allelic gene controlling the same trait. The gene that suppresses said to be epistatic and the gene which remain suppressed is hypostatic. It is also called non-allelic interaction.

Epigenesis: The development of organism like plant and animal from an spore or egg through a series of processes in which undifferentiated cell masses differentiated into organs and organ system.

Euploid: A cell or an organism in which the chromosome number is an exact multiple of the basic number of the concerned species.

F_1 generation: 'F' stands for filial meaning son. F_1 means first filial generation; the progeny obtained by crossing or mating between two individuals.

Factor: Unit of heredity which is responsible for inheritance and appearance of characters. Mendel used term 'factor' for 'gene'.

Fixative: The chemicals used for killing, preserving and fixing plant / animal tissues and specimens in such a way that they retain their original shape, size and structure for a long time.

Gamete: These are reproductive cells that join together to form a new cell called a zygote during sexual reproduction.

Gene: A segment of DNA which specify a single polypeptide or an RNA molecule.

Genetics: The collective study of heredity and variation of inherited characters. Term genetics was coined by W. Bateson in 1905.

Gene interaction: The phenomenon of two or more gene affecting the expression of each other in various ways in the development of single character of an organism is known as gene interaction.

Genome: A complete set of chromosome of a diploid species; all the members of genome are distinct from each other.

Genotype: Genetic constitution of an organism for a particular character.

Germplasm: The hereditary materials transmitted from parents to progeny through germ cell.

Gynandromorph: An individual in which a part of body is male, while the rest of it is female.

Hemizygous: A diploid organism having only one copy of a gene in place of normal two.

Heredity: The process in which traits are passed from parents to offspring.

Heterozygous: A condition in which alleles of a pair have dissimilar effect then individual said to be heterozygous. It produces two different kinds of gametes. Genotype for heterozygous possess both dominant and recessive alleles. For example- Ss

Holandric gene: A gene carried in the Y chromosome and only male to male transmission; confined to male sex only.

Haploid: A cell or an organism having the gametic chromosome number.

Histone: The proteins associated with chromatin in eukaryotes.

Homeologous chromosome pairing: The pairing of chromosomes that are very similar to both gene content and order (differing in their respective DNA content).

Homozygous: A condition in which alleles of a pair have similar effect then individual said to be homozygous. It produces only one type of gamete. Genotype for homozygous possess either dominant or recessive, but never both the alleles. For example- SS or ss.

Homologous chromosome: The chromosomes which pairs regularly and freely with each other during meiosis; there are identical gene content.

Homologous pairing: Pairing of chromosome that are identical with respect to both gene content and order.

Hybrid: The progeny obtained by crossing two individuals having different genotypes.

Hybridization: The process of crossing of two genetically different parents for particular traits.

Hypo-aneuploid: The loss of one or few chromosome in the normal disomic of the species (not a multiple of the basic number, x).

Hyper-aneuploid: The gain of one or few chromosome in the normal disomic of the species.

Incomplete linkage: Linkage between genes that exhibit some crossing over; intermediate in its effects between independent assortment and complete linkage. In this case, recombinant types are recovered with parental type in test cross progeny.

Inhibitory gene action: In this case, a dominant allele at one locus can mask the expression of both (dominant and recessive) alleles at second locus. This is also known as inhibitory gene interaction.

Interference: The occurrence of crossing over in one region of a chromosome interferes with its occurrence in the neighbouring segments called inference.

Intra-generic recombination: Crossing over takes place within a gene.

Inter-generic recombination: Crossing over takes place between two different genes only.

Interkinesis: The stage between the two meiotic divisions is called interkinesis and is generally short lived.

Interphase: The stage of cell cycle in which nucleus of cell is not undergoing division; a period of active protein and DNA synthesis.

Inversion: Rotation of a segment of chromosome by 180^0 so that the gene represent reverse order.

Jumping gene: Genes which keep on changing their position on the chromosome of a genome. Such gene has been reported in maize.

Karyokinesis: The division of nucleus.

Karyotype: The chromosome of a cell arranged according to their length.

Lethal gene: A gene which causes death of all those individuals that carry it in homozygous condition. It may be dominant or recessive.

Limit of resolution: The main distance between two visible bodies at which they can be seen as separate or not in contact with each other.

Linkage: The tendency of two or more genes to stay together during inheritance is known as linkage and it is the consequence of the concerned genes being located in the same chromosome.

Linkage group: All the genes located on particular chromosome, form a linkage group. The number of linkage group correspondent to the number of haploid chromosomes found in a species.

Linkage map: A linear map of the genes showing linkage with each other, it depicts the sequence in which genes are located in the chromosome as well as the frequency of recombination between the adjacent genes. Linkage map was first developed by A. Strutvent.

Magnification: Degree of enlargement, number of times, the length and diameter of an object is multiplied.

Male sterility: The condition in which male organs are absent or non-functional is in bisexual flower known as male sterility.

Map unit: A map unit is that distance in a chromosome, which permits one percent recombination (crossing over) between two linked genes. A map unit is also called a centi-Morgan (cM) or Morgan unit.

Meiosis: A type of cell division in which the number of chromosomes is halved (from diploid to haploid) in the daughter cells, i.e., the gametes. It occurs in cell that produce gametes in sexually reproducing organisms.

Metaphase: The stage during cell division after prophase and before anaphase, the chromosomes are thick, short and distinct from each other.

Microscope: An optical instrument consisting of a lens or combination of lenses for making enlarged images of minute objects.

Microscopy: The science of investigating small objects using such an instrument i.e. microscope is called microscopy.

Mitosis: A process of cell duplication, or reproduction, during which one cell gives rise to two genetically identical daughter cells.

Monohybrid cross: A cross is made between two true-breeding parents differing for a single trait, producing an F_1 generation. Monohybrid cross was first produced in pea by Mendel to explain the "Law of segregation".

Monoploid: An individual having one copy of a single genome; haploid from a diploid species.

Monosomy: An individual having one chromosome less than normal somatic complement of the species.

Multiple allele: More than two alternative form of a gene that occupy the same locus of homologous chromosome.

Multiple crossing over: Occurrence of more than two crossing overs between non-sister chromatids of homologous chromosomes is known as multiple crossing over. However, the frequency of such type of crossing over is extremely low.

Mutable gene: Gene which exhibit higher mutation rate than others. E.g. White eye gene in drosophila.

Mutation: A sudden and heritable change in the characteristics of an organism.

Mutator gene: A gene which enhance the natural mutation rate of other genes in the same genome. E.g. Dotted gene in maize.

Muton: It is the smallest element within a gene, which can give rise to a mutant phenotype or mutation. This indicates that part of a gene can mutate or change.

Non-sister chromatid: Either one of the two chromatids of paired homologous chromosomes.

Nuclear inheritance: The inheritance of genes presents on the chromosome to offspring's is governed by nuclear genes. It follows the Mendelian inheritance.

Nucleoplasm: A highly viscous liquid contained within the nucleus that surrounds the chromosomes and other sub-nuclear organelles.

Nucleosome: A bead like structure of chromatic fibres; composed of histone octamer (H_2A, H_2B, H_3, H_4 x 2) and 146 bp of DNA.

Nucleoside: The pentose sugar and nitrogenous base constitute a nucleoside.

Nucleotide: The unit of DNA which contains one molecule of each phosphate, pentose sugar and nitrogenous base.

Nullisomic: An individual having one chromosome pair less than the normal somatic complement of the species.

Operon: A group of structural genes whose transmission is regulated by a set of a regulator gene, a promoter and an operator.

Oligogenic trait: The traits which are governed by two or few genes; each gene have major effect.

Phenocopy: If different genotypes are present in different environmental condition, then they produce same phenotype. These genotypes are said to be phenocopy of each other.

Phenotype: External or morphological appearance of an organism for a character.

Plasma genes: Genes that are found in the cytoplasm in mitochondria and chloroplast.

Pleiotropy: A single gene affecting more than one character.

Pollen: Pollen in seed-bearing plants, is the gametophyte producing male gamete.

Polygenic trait: The traits governed by several genes which have cumulative or minor effects.

Polymeric gene action: Two dominant non-allelic genes have similar effect when they are separate but produce enhanced effect when they come together.

Principles of independent assortment: It states that alleles of different genes assort independently of one another during gamete formation.

Principles of segregation: Its first principle of Mendel, which states that two alleles of a gene remain separate and do not contaminate each other in the F_1. At the time of gamete formation in F_1 the two alleles separate and pass into different gametes.

Probability: The chance or likelihood of the occurrence of an event.

Prophase: The first stage of cell division in which chromosomes become shorter and thicker and are visible double stranded.

Protein: Protein is nitrogenous organic compound composed of one or more long chains of amino acids and are an essential part of all living organisms.

Protoplasm: The colourless, translucent, odourless and polyphasic fluid comprising the living part of cell.

Pseudo gene: There are some DNA sequences, especially in eukaryotes, which are non-functional or defective copies of normal genes. These sequences do not have any function. Such DNA sequences or genes are known as pseudogenes.

Punnet square: A Punnett square is a grid system that can be set up and used to predict the possible outcomes that may result from the mating process between two individuals, when their genotypes are known. Each cell within the square is representative of one possible genotypic outcome for any offspring.

Purine: Nitrogen containing bases, which consist of double ring structure of nitrogenous bases (adenine and guanine).

Pyrimidine: Nitrogen containing bases, which consist of single ring structure of nitrogenous bases (thymine, cytosine and uracil)

Quasi-diploid: It is also called monosomic-trisomic (2n-1+1, AABCCC) where the chromosome number of the individual is diploid, but the individual is, in fact, aneuploid since it is monosomic for one chromosome and trisomic for the other chromosome at the same time.

Recessive allele: An allele which is incapable of expressing itself phenotypically in the heterozygous state.

Recon: Recons are the regions (units) within a gene between which recombinations can occur, but the recombination cannot occur within a recon.

Replication: The process by which a double-stranded DNA molecule is copied to produce two identical DNA molecules.

Resolution: The ability to reveal closely adjacent structural details as separate and distinct.

Reverse transcription: Synthesis of DNA using RNA as a template; catalysed by reverse transcriptase.

RNA: Ribose nucleic acid; a polynucleotide having ribose as the pentose sugar and ordinary uracil in the place of thymine.

Sat-DNA: In genomic DNA; a narrow peak on a density gradient, representing many tandem repeats or identical short sequence.

Self-incompatibility: The inability of fully functional pollen grains to effect fertilization and seed set on self-pollination.

Self-pollination: The transfer of pollen grains from anther to stigma of same flower of a plant.

Sex index ratio: The ratio of number of X-chromosome to number of set of autosomes.

Sex influenced trait: Genes whose expression depend on the sex of individual. E.g. Gene for baldness in human.

Sex limited trait: A character whose expression is limited in one sex only.

Sex linkage: When the gene of somatic characters are present on allosome in place of autosome is termed as sex linked gene and such phenomenon is known as sex linkage.

Single crossing over: It refers to the formation of single chiasma between non-sister chromatids of homologous chromosomes. It involves two linked genes (Two point test cross).

Sister chromatid: The identical copies (chromatids) formed by the DNA replication of a chromosome, with both copies joined together by a common centromere.

Somatic cell: Any cell of an living organism, excluding the germ cell.

Spindle fibre: The strand like fibre or filament that form during cell division to separate sister chromatids between daughter cells.

Split gene: A gene having non-functional part (intron) along with functional part (exon) is known as split gene. The intervening sequence do not code for amino acids.

Stain: The chemicals which react with the components of the cell to give the component a particular colour for microscopic examination. Stains give the tissues a distinctive colour.

Synapsis: The process in which two homologous chromosomes come in close proximity with one another during prophase I of meiosis, resulting in the formation of bivalent.

Telophase: The final stage of mitosis, and a reversal of many of the processes observed during prophase.

Telomere: The terminal end of a chromosome consists of repetitive nucleotide sequences, which protects the end of the chromosome from deterioration or from fusion with neighbouring chromosomes.

Test cross: It is a type of backcross in which F_1 progeny is crossed with its phenotypically recessive parent. It is used to determine whether the individuals of the F_1 exhibiting dominant character are homozygous or heterozygous.

Tetrasomic: A cell of an organism having one chromosome pair in addition to the normal somatic compliment of a species.

Transcription: The process of making an RNA copy of a gene sequence in the nucleus of cell.

Transition: The substitution in a DNA or an RNA molecule of a purine by another purine or of a pyrimidine by another pyrimidine; lead to a point mutation.

Translation: The process in which ribosomes in the cytoplasm or ER synthesize proteins in the cytoplasm of cell.

Translocation: The integration of a segment of one chromosome into the non-homologous chromosome.

Transversion: The substitution of a purine by pyrimidine or vice versa.

Trans phase linkage: Arrangement of a dominant and recessive allele for two traits are on the same chromosome is known as trans-phase.

Trisomy: An organism having one extra chromosome in addition to the normal somatic complement (2n+1).

Univalent: A chromosome that isn't paired or united with its homologous chromosome during synapsis.

Wobble hypothesis: It state that the first two bases of a codon pair accordingly to the normal base pairing rules with the last two bases of anticodon. Base-pairing at the third position of a codon is wobble (non-Watson-Crick base pairing).

X-linked gene: Gene for somatic characters are located on X-chromosome. It is also called diandric sex-linked gene.

Y-linked gene: Gene for somatic characters are located on Y-chromosome. It is also called holandric gene.

Y-chromosome: Sex chromosome contains some specific gene, which triggers embryonic development as a male.

Zygote: The fusion of one male and one female gamete results in fertilized egg cell known as zygote. It has 2n chromosome complement.

Chapter 1

Study of Simple Microscope

Objectives

- To study working principles of simple microscope
- Study different parts of simple microscope

Introduction

This is the first ever microscope. It was founded by Leeuwenhock in 17th century. He combined a convex lens with a specimen holder, for seeing the magnified images of small objects. It looks like a magnifying glass because it has the capacity to magnify between 200 and 300 times. A simple microscope is a small focal lens used to view the magnified images of small objects. It is just like a hand lens and glass with relatively lower magnification power.

Principle of Simple Microscope

This microscope works on the principle that when a small object is placed within its focus, a virtual, erect and magnified image of the object is formed at the minimum distance of distinct vision from the eye held close to the lens (Fig 1).

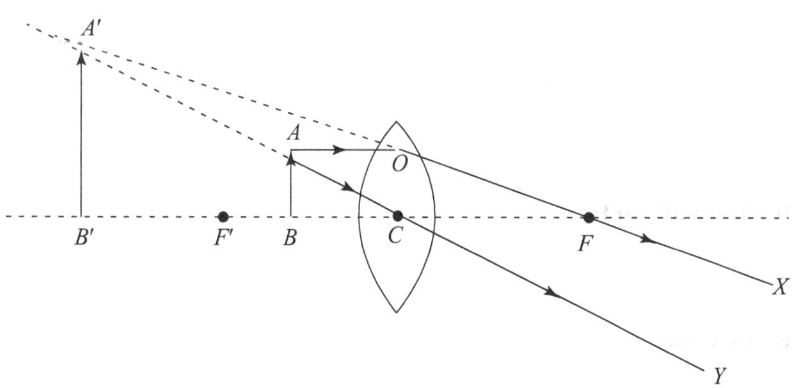

Fig. 1. Ray diagram of simple microscope

Magnification of Simple Microscope

The magnifying power of a simple microscope is given by:

$$M = 1 + D/F$$

Where,

D = least distance of distinct vision

F = focal length of the convex lens

The focal length of the convex lens should be small because smaller the focal length of the lens, greater will be its magnifying power.

A simple microscope's maximum magnification is about 10, which means that by using the simple microscope of maximum magnification, the object will appear 10 times larger.

Parts of a Simple Microscope

The parts of a simple microscope are of two categories as follows:

(i) Mechanical parts

(ii) Optical parts

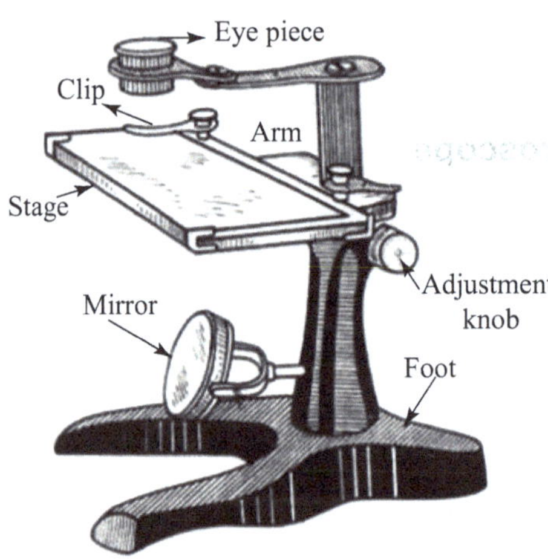

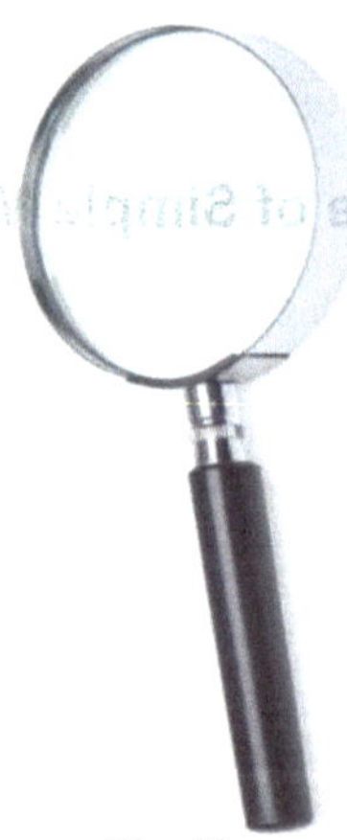

Hand lens

(i) Mechanical parts

These parts support the optical components and help to focus the object in their adjustment. The following components are included:

1. Base or Foot

It is the base component of the simple microscope in horse-shoe-shaped and oval form. This is made up of heavy material. It gives supports to other microscopic sections.

2. Metal Stand
It is fitted with a heavy base plate and a vertical hollow cylindrical rod that provides support and stability for other microscope parts.

3. Stage
It is a metal plate fitted to the vertical rod that is rectangular. It has a central hole from below for light to pass. The slide with the specimen to be observed is kept on the stage, so that the specimen only remains on the central hole. Some microscopes have a couple of slanting wings that project on both sides of the stage. They provide hand-held support for object manipulation.

4. Vertical Limb
The short and movable rod is fitted in the hollow tube of the stand. The limb can be moved up and down by means of the adjustment screw.

5. Folder Arm
It is a horizontal movable arm. Out of two, one of its end is attached with vertical limb and other end is attached with lens. It can be moved up and down as well as left and right.

6. Clips
Clips are two in number and fitted on the stage. These clips are used to kept the slides in desired position.

7. Adjustment Screw
It is a screw used to adjust the vertical limb upwards or downwards.

(ii) Optical parts

These parts involve the transmission of light through the object (specimen) and the magnification of its size. The optical components are as follows.

1. Mirror
Using a frame, a Plano-convex mirror is fitted to the vertical rod below the stage. It focuses on the object to be observed with the surrounding light.

2. Lens
Using a frame, a biconvex lens is attached above the stage to the vertical rod. It magnifies the object's size and by keeping the eye above it, the enlarged virtual image formed is observed. The lens can be moved up and down by the frame for proper focusing.

Utility of simple microscope

- It is used to study of microscopic study of algae, fungi and biological specimen.
- To see the magnified view of different particles of different types of soils.

Important terminology

Microscopy: The science of investigating small objects using such an instrument i.e. microscope is called microscopy.

Magnification: Degree of enlargement, number of times, the length and diameter of an object is multiplied.

Resolution: The ability to reveal closely adjacent structural details as separate and distinct.

Limit of resolution: The main distance between two visible bodies at which they can be seen as separate or not in contact with each other. .

INTEXT QUESTIONS

1. Define the terms
(i) Simple microscope ....

....

....

....

....

....

(ii) Focal length ....

....

....

....

....

....

(iii) Enlist the parts of simple microscope...

....

....

....

....

....

(iv) Formula of magnification of simple microscope ....

....

....

....

....

....

(v) Draw the diagram of simple microscope and indicate different parts.

....

....

....

....

....

....

....

....

....

....

....

....

....

....

....

....

....

....

....

....

Chapter 2

Study of Compound Microscope

Objectives

- To study working principles of compound microscope
- Study different parts of compound microscope

Introduction

A compound microscope is an optical instrument consisting of two short focal-length convex lenses that are used to observe the highly magnified images of small objects by naked eyes. The compound microscope is capable of magnifying up to 1000 the image of a small object by complex system of lens arrangement. The working distance varies from 0.14 to 4 mm. Compound microscopes generally require the sample to be seen to be sufficiently thin, or translucent, to allow the light to pass. Such microscopes provide high magnification, but the view is two-dimensional.

Principle of Compound Microscope

A compound microscope works on the principle that when a small object to be magnified is placed just beyond the focus of its objective lens, a virtual, inverted and highly magnified image of the object is formed at a minimum distance from the eye near the piece of the eye.

It has a series of two lenses; (i) the objective lens near the object to be observed; and (ii) the eye lens or eye piece through which the image is viewed by the eye. The specimen must be thin transparent for light to pass through it easily.

The objective lens creates an object's magnified 'real image' (first image). The eye-piece lens magnifies this image again in order to obtain a magnified 'virtual image' (final image) that can be seen through the eye-piece (Fig. 2.1 and 2.2). As light passes directly through the two lenses from the source to the eye, the field of vision is illuminated brightly.

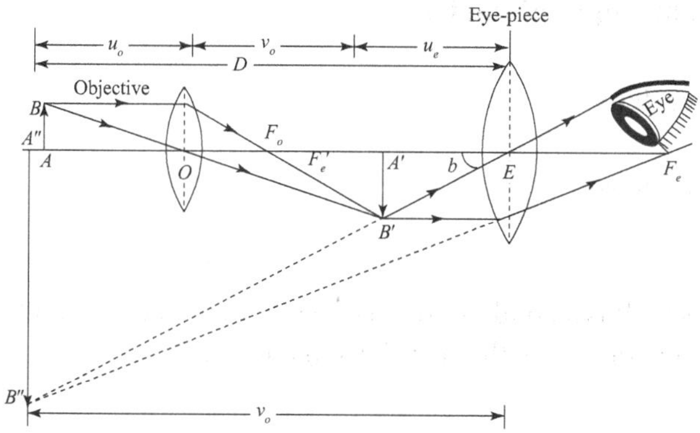

Fig. 2.1 Ray diagram of compound microscope

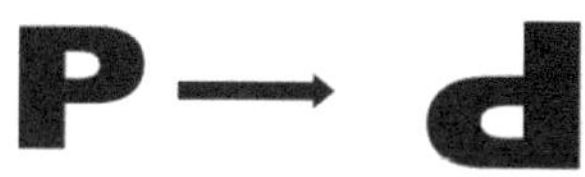

Fig. 2.2 The letter P through compound microscope

Magnification of compound microscope

The magnification of compound microscope is given by:

$$M = D/F_o \times L/F_e$$

Where,

D = Least distance of distinct vision (25 cm)
L = Length of the microscope tube
F_o = Focal length of the objective lens
F_e = Focal length of the eye-piece lens

Parts of a Compound Microscope

The compound microscope consists of two main parts.

1. Lens systems (optical parts)
2. Mechanical parts.

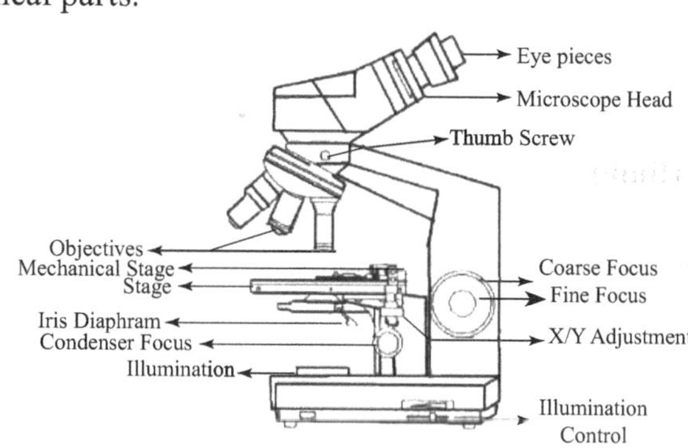

1. Lens systems (optical parts)

There are three types of lens systems.

(a) **Eye piece lens**: It lies on the top of the body tube. They are usually magnified by 5X, 10X, 15X.

(b) **Objective lens**: It is attached to the nose piece. They are of various magnifications for oil immersion, such as 10X (low power) and other high power (40X) and 100X. The most widely used objective lens is 10X.

(c) **Condenser**: It is a condensed lens system that receives light rays from the mirror and converges them at the stage level.

(d) **Mirror**: Under the stage it's mobile, detachable and fitted. Its one side is concave and other side is plane or flat surface. The diaphragm reflects light upward.

2. Mechanical parts

They include the following components:

(a) **Base**: This is the microscope's lowest part. It bears the weight. It's in the form of 'U' or triangular. It supports the microscope's body.

(b) **Body tube**: It is a microscope body which consists of a tube called the body tube. It can move up and down in the vertical direction. It carries two lenses, in other words, eye piece and objective at appropriate distance.

(c) **Inclination joint**: It joins the microscope lower and upper parts. You can tilt the upper part of the microscope to suit the observer's eye level.

(d) **Fine adjustment knob**: It is small - sized screw. It is mounted on the body tube. It moves up and down the body tube and it can make precise focusing.

(e) **Coarse adjustment knob**: It is attached to the body tube, which for focusing can be moved up and down.

(f) **Stage with clips**: It is a platform with a circular hole in the center on which the slide is placed and the clips are fixed.

(g) **Nose-piece:** It is a circular structure of metal attached under the body tube. It is a rotating part to adjust the objectives. There are three or four objectives fitted in the nose–piece with lens.

(h) **Body arm (limb)**: It supports the body tube. It is usually curved. It is used to hold the microscope.

(i) **Diaphragm**: It is installed below the stage. It controls the quantity of light incident on the lens.

Working of Compound Microscope

First of all, look at the eye-piece and adjust the mirror to allow enough light to reach the microscope. Now make sure the stage, mirror, lenses, and slides don't have any dirt. In the center of the stage, position the slide. Place the clips on both slide corners to stop it from moving. Now turn the nose piece and align the low power objective in line with the object to be seen in the slide. Now move or adjust the rough adjustment knob up or down to get the slide in view. Step up or down the fine adjustment knob to sharpen the image as much as possible. (Observe all material details under low power and draw the diagram). Now turn the nose piece and bring the high power objective in line with the object. Use the fine adjustment knob again to sharpen and clear the image of the object as possible. Observe the details of the material under high power and draw the diagram. Do not use coarse adjustment knob during studying under high power. It may break the slide.

Precautions when using a microscope

(a) Place the microscope in highest disseminated light.
(b) First fix the low observation power.
(c) Always use a muslin cloth or soft handkerchief to clean the lenses or mirror.
(d) Slide is supposed to be dry and clean.
(e) To adjust proper light, use diaphragm.
(f) Do not touch with your hands the lens, objective, mirror or diaphragm.
(g) Never leave after use a slide on the stage.
(h) Use both hands to hold the microscope.

Difference between simple and compound microscope

Simple microscope	Compound microscope
Simple microscope is actually a convex lens of small focal length, which is used to see the magnified image of small objects. It is also known as magnifying glass.	Compound microscope is an optical instrument consisting of two convex lenses of short focal length which is used for highly magnified image of small objects.
It consist one convex lens.	It consist two convex lens.
Magnification power is 10.	Magnification power is 1000.
Mirror is concave type.	Mirror is plain at one side and concave at other side.
No adjusting magnification.	We can adjust magnification.
Light source is natural.	Illuminator type.
Condenser lens is absent.	Condenser lens is present.

INTEXT QUESTIONS

1. Define the terms

(i) Compound Microscope ....

....

....

....

....

....

(ii) Objective Lens ....

....

....

....

....

....

(iii) Eyepiece Lens ....

....

....

....

....

....

2. Enlist the parts of Compound Microscope

....

....

....

....

....

3. Formula of Magnification of Compound Microscope

....

....

....

....

....

4. Draw the diagram of Compound Microscope

....

....

....

....

....

5. Draw the ray diagram of Compound Microscope

....

....

....

....

....

6. Complete the following chart

PARTS	FUNCTION
Eyepiece lens	
Objective lens	
Arm	
Diaphragm	
Fine adjustment	
Coarse adjustment	

Chapter 3

Study of Fixatives and Stains

Objectives

- Differentiate between fixatives and stains.
- Describe methods of staining.
- List the commonly used fixatives and stains and their composition.
- Describe the uses of above mentioned solutions and stains.

Introduction

Every time a part of an organism is removed, the action of bacteria will soon disintegrate, dry or putrefy it. They must be kept as close to normal as possible or in other words preserved and fixed in order to study these. Chemicals are required in many practical of Biology. Some of these chemicals preserve and specifically colour certain cell parts while others are used as solutions. You will learn about certain fixatives (preservatives) and stains in this chapter.

1. Fixatives (Preservatives)

Fixatives are the chemicals used for killing, preserving and fixing plant / animal tissues and specimens in such a way that they retain their original shape, size and structure for a long time. The tissue removed from the body must be penetrated quickly by a fixative. Fixing also makes the material fit for staining. Fixatives also harden and prevent the tissues from decaying. The latter is usually washed in running water after the material is fixed and then kept in an appropriate preservative.

Objectives of fixation

(a) To preserve tissues as close as possible to their living conditions
(b) Hardening tissues
(c) Preventing tissues from altering their form and size during handling
(d) Preventing autolysis and bacterial attack
(e) Transparent staining of parts thereafter
(f) Improving the optical distinction of cells and tissues

Popular Fixative Solutions

A large number of chemicals such as ethyl alcohol, formalin, acetic acid, chloroform, mercuric chloride, chromic acid, picric acid, osmic acid, etc. are used as fixatives for anatomical studies either individually or in combinations. Formalin and formalin-aceto-alcohol (FAA) are among these most commonly used in anatomy. Some of the fixatives are given below along with their composition:

A. Formalin and Formalin-Aceto-Alcohol (FAA)

It is a very good fixative and without any harm, tissues can be left in it for a long time. A number of variations were suggested, but the standard proportions are:

a. Composition of FAA	
50 % Alcohol	90 ml
40 % Formaldehyde	5 ml
Glacial acetic acid	5 ml

b. Composition of FAA	
50 % Alcohol	85 ml
40 % Formaldehyde	5 ml
Glacial acetic acid	10 ml

The lower alcohol content is more appropriate for sensitive materials such as bryophytes. It is better to reduce the amount of acetic acid for hard and woody materials and to increase the amount of formalin, i.e. use the second mixture, as formalin penetrates more slowly. The material can be left almost indefinitely in FAA without any significant damage. It's a universal standard fixative. For cells and tissues, it is a good preservative.

B. Bouin's fluid

Pol Andre Bouin introduced the Bouin's Fluid in the year 1897 as a distinguished French scientist. It is yellow in colour and penetrates rapidly in the tissues, for making histological preparation. It is used to fix tissue from plants and animals. For a long time, the materials treated with it may be stored.

Composition of Bouin's fluid	
Saturaded aqueous picric acid	75 ml
Formaline (40 % Formaldehyde)	25 ml
Glacial acetic acid	5 ml

C. Farmer's fluid or Carnoy's fluid I (1886)

It is prepared by mixing glacial acetic acid and absolute ethyl alcohol in 1:3 ratio. Alcohol causes shrinkage of protoplasm whereas acetic acid causes its swelling, therefore this combination keeps the protoplasm intact. Plant maternal is kept in this solution for 1–4 hrs. Solution should be prepared just before its use. This fixative is also used for animal and human materials.

Composition of Carnoy's fluid I	
Absolute alcohol	30 ml
Glacial acetic acid	10 ml

D. Carnoy's fluid II (1886)

It is prepared by mixing glacial acetic acid, chloroform and absolute ethyl alcohol in the proportion of 1:3:6. Plant material (flower buds) is kept in this solution for 1–4 hrs. It penetrates rapidly and gives excellent nuclear fixation. Mitotic chromosomes of soft material like root tips, which need lesser time for fixations, respond well with these mixture. The tissues are transferred to 95 per cent or absolute alcohol after fixation.

Composition of Carnoy's fluid II	
Absolute alcohol	60 ml
Chloroform	30 ml
Glacial acetic acid	10 ml

E. Clarke's Fluid

J.L. Clarke introduced the Clarke's Fluid in 1851 and this fixative was named after him eventually. The fixative of the Clarke was initially implemented for the nervous system. It was the first histological fixative to have a formula published. The product was 3 components of not less than 95% or 96% alcohol and 1 component of pure acetic acid. It preserve nucleic acids but extracts lipids.

Composition of Clarke's fluid	
Ethanol (absolute)	75 ml
Acetic acid glacial	25 ml

F. Zenker's Fluid

Albert von Zenker introduced the Zenker's fluid. This is a fast-acting fixative for animal tissues that contains mercury chloride, potassium dichromate, sodium sulphate, water, and acetic acid. It's a good fixative routine that gives relatively quick and even penetration. It provides excellent nuclear preservation but owing to the existence of acetic acid it lyses red blood cells.

Composition of Zenker's fluid	
Distilled water	950 ml
Mercuric chloride	50 g
Potassium dichromate	25 g
Glacial acetic acid	50 ml

2. Stains

Stains are the chemicals which react with the components of the cell to give the component a particular colour for microscopic examination. Stains give the tissues a distinctive color. Different stains differently colour varying cell or tissue components. This makes it more comfortable for the microscopic analysis. These dyes may be synthetic chemicals or obtained from plants or animals e.g. carmine is derived from the cochineal insect. There are different stains for study of different biological materials. Staining can be done in several ways:

(a) ***Single staining*:** Where only one stain is used giving a single colour to the tissue e.g., Acetocarmine stains both the nucleus and the cytoplasm pink.

(b) ***Double staining*:** Where two stains are used, each stains a specific area or the particular cell organelle e.g., Methyl green which stains nucleus green is used with Pyronin which stains the cytoplasm pink.

(c) ***Multiple staining*:** More than two stains are used in the preparation of slide of tissue or organelle. Each stain will colour only the specific organelle of the cell e.g., Triple Mallory stain.

(d) ***Vital staining*:** Stains such as the Janus Green B which stains mitochondria is used to colour living cells. Such stains which do not kill the cell, do not require prior fixation and impart colour to a specific part are termed vital stains (vita = live).

Two main types of stains are used-

(a) **Temporary stains:** whose colour fades or which gradually damages the sections.

Examples: Methylene blue, Chlor-zinc-iodine solution (Schult's solution), Chlorazol black, Phloroglucin and conc. HCl, Sudan IV, Iodine with potassium iodide, Eosin etc.

(b) **Permanent stains:** whose colour lasts for many years.

Permanent staining is always accompanied by complete dehydration and clearing followed by mounting in Canada balsam or euparal etc.

Some commonly used stains are given below:

i. **Leishman's Stain:** It is a readymade double stain, used for staining blood films. It gives blue colour to the nucleus and pink to the cytoplasm. For good results this stain is kept in dark coloured bottle. With this dye, stain red RBCs, stain blue nuclei of WBCs, and stain violet platelets. Dissolving the leishman stain powder in methyl alcohol will prepare this stain and leave it to mature for 48 hours.

Composition	
Leishman stain powder	15 g
Methyl alcohol (solvent)	100 ml

ii **Safranin:** It is used as a general stain for plant tissues. The stain may be prepared both in water as well as in 90% alcohol depending on the requirement. It is a synthetic dye which gives pink or red colour to the object stained. It is used to stain lignified tissues, cutinised tissues and nucleus. This stain is prepared by dissolving safranin powder to the alcohol.

Composition	
Safranin powder	1 g
Distilled water	100 ml

iii. **Acetocarmine:** It is mainly used to stain chromosomes of cell dark red. It commonly used to study chromosomes and cell division. This stain is prepared by boiling in the combination of acetic acid and water by dissolving carmine powder. On refrigeration, add a couple of drops of ferric acetate. Filter and store in a bottle of darkness.

Composition	
Glacial acetic acid	45 ml
Carmine powder	2 g
Distilled water	55 ml

iv. **Methylene blue:** This stain may be used both as aqueous or alcoholic stain. It is a basic stain and so mainly stains acidic parts such as DNA of the nucleus and fungal bodies. Methylene blue is a vital stain. Composition of aqueous and alcoholic methylene blue stain is:

(a) **Aqueous Methylene blue:** The stain is dissolved in distilled water

(b) **Alcoholic Methylene blue:** This stain is prepared by adding 30 ml of saturated alcoholic solution of methylene blue (0.3 gm of it to 30 ml of 95% ethyl alcohol) in 100 ml of distilled water.

Composition of Aqueous Methylene blue	
Methylene blue	100 mg
Distilled water	100 ml

Alcoholic Methylene blue	
Methylene blue	0.3 g
95% Ethyl alcohol	30 ml
Distilled water	100 ml

v. **Eosin:** Sometimes a 1% aqueous eosin solution is used. It provides the fabric an overall yellowish appearance. It is used as a stain of cytoplasm. This is ready by dissolving the distilled water with eosin dust.

Composition	
Eosin powder	1 g
Distilled water	100 ml

INTEXT QUESTIONS

1. Define the terms

(i) Fixative ....

....

....

....

....

....

(ii) Stain ....

....

....

....

....

....

2. Enlist the different types of Fixatives..

....

....

....

....

....

3. State the composition of Carnoy's fluid and Iodine solution. ....

....

....

....

....

....

4. Write down the importance of fixative and stain. ....

....

....

....

....

....

5. Write the full form of F.A.A. ....

....

....

....

....

....

6. Mention the use of

(i) Safranin ....

....

....

....

....

....

(ii) Leishman's stain ....

....

....

....

....

....

Chapter 4

Preparation of Onion Root Tip Slides Showing Various Stages of Mitosis Cell Division Using Squash Processing Technique

Objectives

- Better understand the process and different stages of mitosis.
- Prepare your own specimens of onion root in which you can visualize all of the stages of mitosis.

Principle

The genetic information of plants, animals and other eukaryotic organisms resides in several (or many) individual DNA molecules, or chromosomes. For example, each human cell possesses 46 chromosomes, while each cell of an onion possesses 8 chromosomes. All cells must replicate their DNA when dividing.

DNA replication in eukaryotes is followed by the process called mitosis which assures that each daughter cell receives one copy of each of the replicated chromosomes. During the process of mitosis, the chromosomes pass through several stages known as prophase, metaphase, anaphase and telophase. The actual division of the cytoplasm is called cytokinesis and occurs during telophase. During each of the preceding stages, particular events occur that contribute to the orderly distribution of the replicated chromosomes prior to cytokinesis.

An onion root tip is a rapidly growing part of the onion and thus many cells will be in different stages of mitosis. The onion root tips can be prepared and squashed in a way that allows them to be flattened on a microscopic slide, so that the chromosomes of individual cells can be observed easily. The super coiled chromosomes during different stages of mitosis present in the onion root tip cells can be visualized by treating with DNA specific stains, like Feulgen stain and Acetocarmine stain.

Materials required

Onion plant with root, acetocarmine stain, 1 N HCl, scissors, forceps, razor blade, spirit lamp, needle, microscopic slides and cover slips, light microscope, incubator, refrigerator, oven, watch plates.

Prepared chemical solutions

Colchicine (0.1%): In 100 ml of distilled water, put 0.1 g of colchicine powder. Before using, shake well. Store in the refrigerator..

Fixative (Carnoy fluid): The Carnoy fluid is formed by blending 1:3 proportion of glacial acetic acid and absolute ethyl alcohol. Before use, prepare fresh. Keep it at room temperature.

HCl (1N): it is prepared by mixing 8.25 ml HCl in 91.75 ml of distilled water. Before use, keep in the oven at 60 °C.

Acetocarmine (2%): Dissolve 2 g of carmine in 100 ml of 45 percent acetic acid prepared by blending 45 ml of glacial acetic acid and 55 ml of distilled water and reflux by mild boiling for about 2 hours. Then store it in a brown dropper bottle in a refrigerator.

Procedure

1. Germination

   The roots are produced at room temperature from onion bulbs in aerated distilled water. Collect vigorously growing 0.5-1.5 cm long, wash, and dry healthy roots 2 or 3 days old.

2. Pre-treatment

   Cut and wash in running tap water fresh young onion root about 0.5–1.5 cm long.

   The washed root tips are pre-treated in a BOD incubator with 0.1 percent colchicine/saturated solution of 8-hydroxyquinoline or bromonapthanile or para-dichlorobenzene or chloral hydrates for 2–3 hours at 25 °C, to increase the number of dividing cells, to induce chromosome and arms condensation and to clarify the cytoplasmic debris.

3. Fixation

   The pretreated roots tips are cleaned and moved to the fixative (Carnoy's fluid) at 25 °C for at least 24 hours, to maintain the cell in normal state.

4. Preservation

   Preserve the tissue at 2–4 °C in 70 percent ethyl alcohol until needed.

5. Hydrolysis

   It is performed to soften the tissue and causes cell and chromosomes scattering. Place one drop of 1N HCL on the root tip and keep it in an oven for 10 minutes at 60 °C. Wash it with the tap water.

6. Squash preparation

   Put the hydrolysed root in 2 percent acetone in a covered watch plate for 10 minutes or until the meristematic part of the root peel is deep red, whereas, the remainder of the portion is lightly stained. Take a drop of acetocarmine on a new slide and softly trimmed the tip of the root. Disposed the lightly stained area of root cap with a blade or needle. Make 3–4 pieces, tease and put under cover slip. Warm the slide gently over the alcohol lamp for about one minute. (Do not allow the slide to get hot to the touch; you don't want to cook either your fingers or the root. Do not let the root dry out). Carefully blot the excess stain with a blotting paper. Squash the slide with your thumb using a firm and even pressure. (Avoid squashing with such force that the cover slip breaks or slides).

7. Observation

   The squashed preparations are observed under compound microscope in 10x objective. Scan and narrow down to a region containing dividing cells and switch to 40x for a better view.

Why use the roots of onion to see mitosis?

- Roots cab easily grow in significant numbers.
- Root tip cells are actively dividing, and therefore many cells will be in mitosis stage.
- Tips can be prepared in a way that allows them to be flattened on microscopes slide ("squashed") so that the chromosomes of individual cells can be observed.
- The chromosomes can be coloured to make them easier to see.

Precautions

1. Use clean slides and coverslips.
2. While fixing the tissues do not leave it in acid for more than the required time.
3. Do not heat the slide. It is only to be warmed.
4. After putting coverslip over stained material, blot off excess stain.
5. Do not allow the slide to dry up.

Stages of mitosis

The process of Mitosis is divided into four stages: Prophase, Metaphase, Anaphase and Telophase as shown in Fig. 1.

Prophase: During this stage, the chromosomes super coil, condense and become visible for first time during the cell cycle. The spindle fibers start forming. The nuclear membrane and nucleolus starts disintegrating.

Metaphase: During this stage, the spindle fibers reach and attach to centromere of each sister chromatids. The chromosomes become arranged on the equatorial plane. The nuclear membrane disintegrates completely.

Anaphase: The shortest stage of mitosis. The centromeres divide, and the sister chromatids of each chromosome are pulled apart - or 'disjoin' - and move to the opposite ends of the cell, pulled by spindle fibres attached to the kinetochore regions. The separated sister chromatids are now referred to as daughter chromosomes. (It is the alignment and separation in metaphase and anaphase that is important in ensuring that each daughter cell receives a copy of every chromosome).

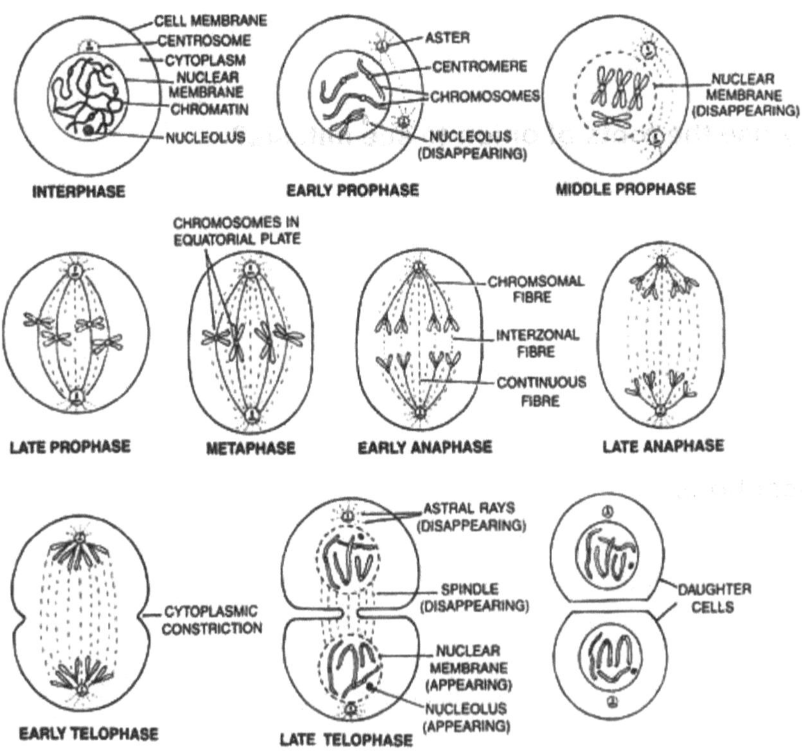

Fig. 1. Diagrammatic representation of different stages of mitotic cell division.

Telophase: The final stage of mitosis, and a reversal of many of the processes observed during prophase. Chromosomes have reached the opposite poles. Nuclear membrane reforms around the chromosomes grouped at either pole of the cell, the chromosomes uncoil and become diffuse, and the spindle fibres disappear.

Cytokinesis: The final cellular division to form two new cells. In plants a cell plate forms along the line of the metaphase plate; in animals there is a constriction of the cytoplasm. The cell then enters interphase - the interval between mitotic divisions.

Biological significance of mitosis

- Mitosis is important for sexual reproduction indirectly.
- It allows the sexually reproducing organism to grow and develop from a single cell into a sexually mature individual.
- This allows organisms to continue reproduce through the generation.
- Repairing and regeneration of damaged tissues in body occur by mitosis.
- Mitosis produces the cells which form new organism in asexual reproduction.
- In mitosis, the heredity material is equally distributed in the daughter cells.
- As there is no recombination in mitosis, the genetic information remains unchanged generation after generation, thus continuity of similar information is ensured from parent to daughter cell.
- It is the only way to increase the cell number without any change in genetic material.

Points to be remember

A. Difference between prophase and telophase

	Prophase		Telophase
1.	Chromatin fibres become condensed	1.	Chromatin fibre become de-condensed.
2.	Nucleolus get disappear.	2.	Nucleolus get reappear.
3.	Nucleus membrane start disappear.	3.	Nucleus membrane reappear.
4.	Chromatin becomes chromosome.	4.	Chromosomes become chromatin.

B. Difference between metaphase and anaphase

	Metaphase		Anaphase
1.	Chromosomes get arranged on equator	1.	The daughter chromosomes start moving towards pole from equator line.
2.	Centromere of chromosomes touches equator line and chromosomal arm faces toward poles.	2.	Chromosomes arranged in such a way that centromere takes the leading position and their arms follows it.
3.	Spindle fibres are attached to kinetochores.	3.	Chromosomes moves towards opposite poles by shortening of spindle fibres.

INTEXT QUESTIONS

1. Find and draw a cell showing each stage of mitosis.

Prophase	Metaphase	Anaphase	Telophase

2. What is a distinguishing visible feature of each stage of mitosis?

Prophase: ....

....

....

....

....

....

Metaphase: ....

....

....

....

....

....

Anaphase: ....

....

....

....

....

....

Telophase: ....

....

....

....

....

....

3. During mitosis, a cell with 42 chromosomes will produce daughter cells with how many chromosomes?

....

....

....

....

....

4. Why metaphase stage of mitosis is best for chromosomal study?

....

....

....

....

....

5. What is the significance of mitotic cell division?

....

....

....

....

....

....

6. Match the following:

	Column I		**Column II**
1.	Prophase	A	Reformation of nucleolus and nuclear membrane
2	Metaphase	B	Nucleolus and nuclear membrane disappear
3	Anaphase	C	Formation of mctaphasc platc
4	Telophase	D	Movement of daughter chromosomes towards poles

7. Label each figure with the stage of mitosis that it represents.

(a) 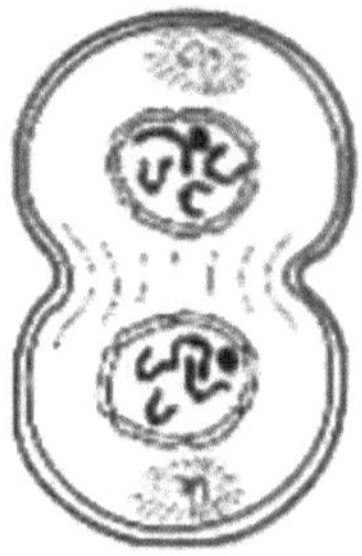

(b) 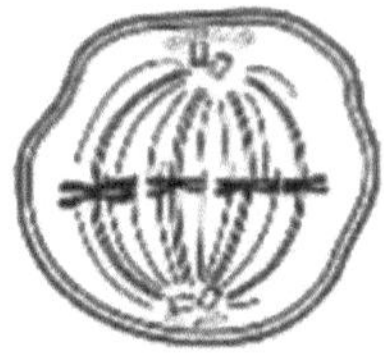

(c) 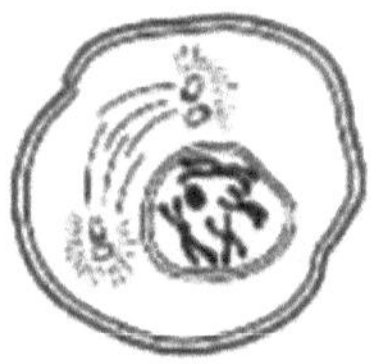

(d) 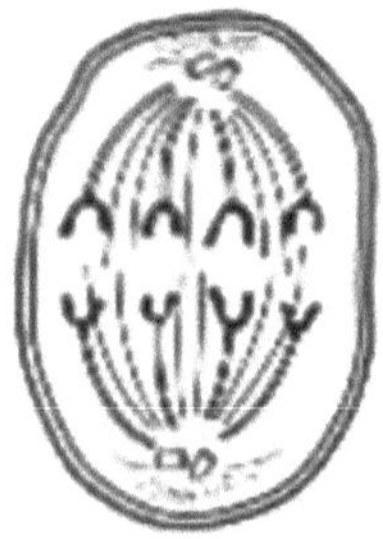

8. Arrange the diagram below shows the stages of mitosis in systematic order. Choose the correct answer.

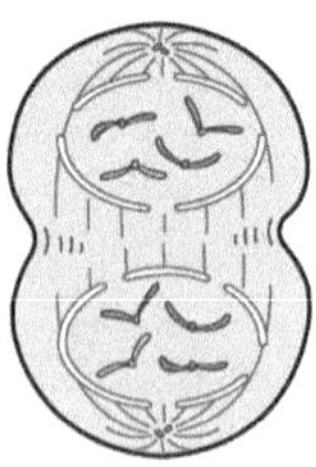

(I)

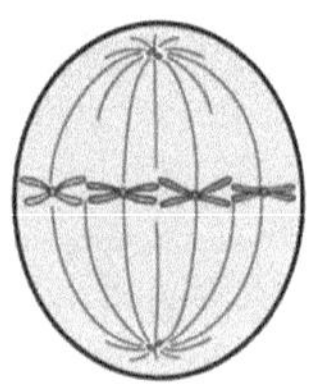

(II)

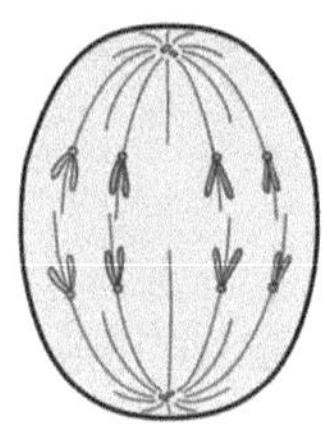

(III)

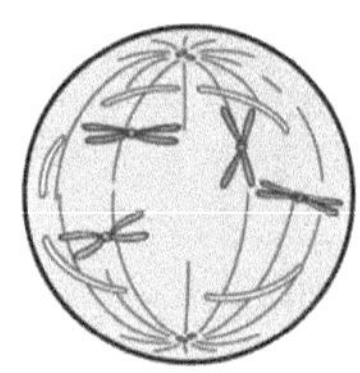

(IV)

(a) I – II – IV – III
(b) III – I – II – IV
(c) IV – II – III – I
(d) IV – III – II – I

Chapter 5

Preparation of Slides Using Flower Bud Showing Various Stages of Meiosis Cell Division

Objectives

- Better understand the process and different stages of meiosis.
- Prepare your own specimens of onion root in which you can visualize all of the stages of meiosis.

Principle

Meiosis is a type of cell division in which the number of chromosomes is halved (from diploid to haploid) in the daughter cells, i.e., the gametes. It occurs in cell that produce gametes in sexually reproducing organisms. The division is completed in two phases, meiosis I and meiosis II. Meiosis I is a reductional division in which the chromosomes of homologous pairs separate from each other. Meiosis II maintain same number of chromosomes, hence, is called as equational division. Stages of meiosis can be observed in a cytological preparation of the pollen mother cells of the anthers of flower buds.

Material required

Flower buds, slides, cover slips, microscope, 0.2–2% acetocarmine stain, needle, forceps, incubator, refrigerator, oven, brush, watch glass, spirit lamp etc.

Procedure

1. **Floral organ collection**

   Meiosis occurs only once in the lifetime in the pollen mother cell. The stage of anthers and time of meiosis of specific species should be known before collection of bulk of the material of studies. Select appropriate flower buds of different size from the inflorescence, starting from the smallest and working up to the largest, until a correct bud having divisional stage is found.

2. **Fixation**

   It is the preservation of all cellular and structural elements in as closely to the natural living conditions as possible. A better fixative is one that least shifts the structure of the cells. The most frequently used fixatives are Carnoy's fluid I and Carnoy's fluid II.

3. **Preservation**

   Preserve the tissue at 2–4 °C in 70 percent ethyl alcohol until needed.

4. **Slide preparation**

   The fixed/ preserved anthers are squashed and teased in an acetocarmine drop of 2%. In the case of large anther, debris should be removed before placing the carmine drop on the material. Leave the material in the stain for 5 minutes. Place a cover slip over them and tap it gently with a needle or pencil. Warm it slightly over the flame of a spirit lamp. Put a piece of blotting paper on the cover slip and apply uniform pressure with your thumb.

5. **Observation**

   Examine the slide under the microscope, search for different stages of meiosis and count the chromosomes/ bivalents along with their characteristic features.

Precautions

(a) Use clean slides and coverslips.

(b) While fixing the tissues do not leave it in acid for more than the required time.

(c) Do not heat the slide. It is only to be warmed.

(d) After putting coverslip over stained material, blot off excess stain.

(e) Do not allow the slide to dry up.

Stages of meiosis

Farmer and Moore suggested the term meiosis. Meiosis usually produces different types of cell. All the four daughter cells formed by meiosis differ genetically from each other and also differ from parent cell. Meiotic events is completed in two phases, meiosis I (reductional division) and meiosis II (equational division).

Meiosis I

Meiosis I separates the pairs of homologous chromosomes. This is a heterotypic or reductional division. It leads to reduction in chromosome numbers. Division of chromosomes are not occur in meiosis I, but only segregation of homologous chromosomes takes place. This division of meiosis consists of the four phases :

1. Prophase I
2. Metaphase I
3. Anaphase I
4. Telophase I

1. Prophase I: Prophase of the first meiotic division is typically longer and more complex when compared to prophase of mitosis. It has been further subdivided into the following five phases based on chromosomal behaviour.

(a) ***Leptotene*:** During leptotene stage the chromosomes become gradually visible under the light microscope. The compaction of chromosomes continues throughout leptotene.

(b) ***Zygotene***: During this stage chromosomes start pairing together and this process of association is called synapsis. Such paired chromosomes are called homologous chromosomes. Electron micrographs of this stage indicate that chromosome synapsis is accompanied by the formation of complex structure called synaptonemal complex. The complex formed by a pair of synapsed homologous chromosomes is called a bivalent or a tetrad. However, these are more clearly visible at the next stage.

(c) ***Pachytene***: During this stage bivalent chromosomes now clearly appears as tetrads. This stage is characterised by the appearance of recombination nodules, the sites at which crossing over occurs between non-sisters chromatids of the homologous chromosomes. Crossing over is the exchange of genetic material between two homologous chromosomes. Recombination between homologous chromosomes is completed by the end of pachytene, leaving the chromosomes linked at the sites of crossing over.

(d) ***Diplotene***: The beginning of diplotene is recognised by the dissolution of the synaptonemal complex and the tendency of the recombined homologous chromosomes of the bivalents to separate from each other except at the sites of crossovers. These X-shaped structures, are called chiasmata.

(e) ***Diakinesis***: The final stage of meiotic prophase I is diakinesis. This is marked by terminalisation of chiasmata. During this phase the chromosomes are fully condensed and the meiotic spindle is assembled to prepare the homologous chromosomes for separation. By the end of diakinesis, the nucleolus disappears and the nuclear envelope also breaks down. Diakinesis represents transition to metaphase.

2. Metaphase I: The bivalent chromosomes align on the equatorial plate. The microtubules from the opposite poles of the spindle attach to the pair of homologous chromosomes.

3. Anaphase I: The homologous chromosomes separate, while sister chromatids remain associated at their centromeres. This stage is characterized by segregation of homologous chromosome. Division of centromere is absent.

4. Telophase I: The nuclear membrane and nucleolus reappear, cytokinesis follows and this is called as dyad of cells. Although in many cases the chromosomes do undergo some dispersion, they do not reach the extremely extended state of the interphase nucleus. The stage between the two meiotic divisions is called **interkinesis** and is generally short lived. Interkinesis is followed by prophase II, a much simpler prophase than prophase I.

Meiosis II

This is a homotypic or equational division. It does not leads to any changes in chromosome numbers. Division of chromosomes and centromere occurs in meiosis II. This division resembles with mitosis, during which both the haploid daughter cells pass through the following stages to form four haploid cells. This division of meiosis consists of the four phases:

1. Prophase II
2. Metaphase II
3. Anaphase II
4. Telophase II

1. Prophase II: Meiosis II is initiated immediately after cytokinesis, usually before the chromosomes have fully elongated. In contrast to meiosis I, meiosis II resembles a normal mitosis. The nuclear membrane disappears by the end of prophase II. The chromosomes again become compact.

2. Metaphase II: At this stage the chromosomes align at the equator and the microtubules from opposite poles of the spindle get attached to the kinetochores of sister chromatids.

3. Anaphase II: It begins with the simultaneous splitting of the centromere of each chromosome (which was holding the sister chromatids together), allowing them to move toward opposite poles.

4. Telophase II: Meiosis ends with telophase II, in which the two groups of chromosomes once again get enclosed by a nuclear envelope; cytokinesis follows resulting in the formation of tetrad of cells i.e., four haploid daughter cells.

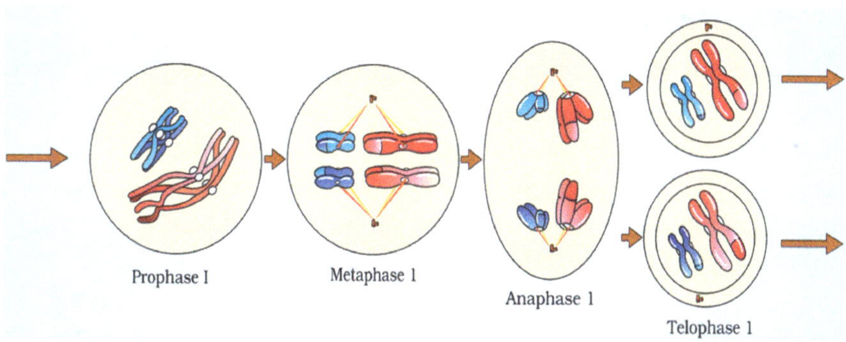

Stages of meiosis-I

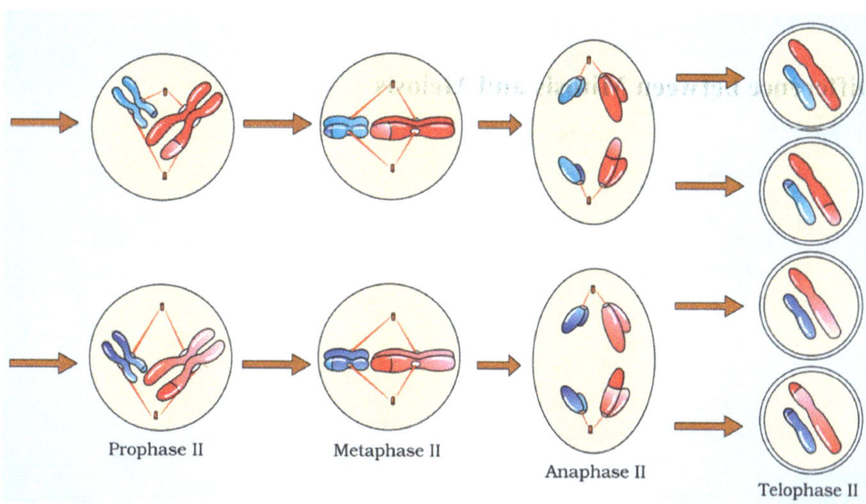

Fig. Diagrammatic representation of difference between mitosis and meiosis

Biological significance of meiosis

- Production of gametes: It is the only process that produce haploid gametes.
- Reduction in chromosome number: It ensures that each gametes has only half the number of chromosomes of the parent cell.
- Maintenance of chromosome number in somatic cell: The conservation of specific chromosome number of each species is achieved across generation in sexually reproducing organism.
- Production of variation: crossing over increases genetic diversity as the genes on the chromosome combine in number of ways. It causes genetic variation in the descendants. It can produce individuals who do not resemble their parents closely. These variations are the causes of evolution.

Difference between Mitosis and Meiosis

S. No.	Mitosis	Meiosis
1.	It occurs continuously in the body or somatic cells.	It occurs in reproductive or germ cells during gametogenesis.
2.	The whole process complete in one sequence or phase after one round of DNA replication.	The whole process complete in two successive divisions which occur one after the other.
3.	The prophase is of short duration and does not include any sub-stage.	The prophase is of longer duration and it includes five sub-stage.
4.	The homologous chromosomes duplicate into two chromatids. The chromatids separate and form new chromosomes.	Out of the two homologous chromosomes only one type of chromosome either maternal or paternal moves to the daughter cells.
5.	No pairing takes place between the homologous chromosomes.	Pairing or synapsis occur between the homologous chromosomes.
6.	Chromosome duplication takes place in the early prophase.	Duplication or splitting of chromosomes takes place in the late prophase.
7.	No crossing over takes place.	Crossing over takes place.
8.	No chiasma formation takes place.	Chiasma formation takes place.
9.	The chromosome number remains the same in the newly formed daughter cells.	Chromosome number is reduced into half in the newly formed daughter cells.
10.	Two daughter cells are formed.	Four daughter cells are formed.
11.	Daughter cells are similar	Daughter cells are dissimilar
12.	Nucleus and cytoplasm divide once.	Nucleus and cytoplasm divide twice.
13.	Synapsis formation do not occur.	Synapsis formation occur.
14.	Chiasmata formation do not takes place.	Chiasmata formation occur.

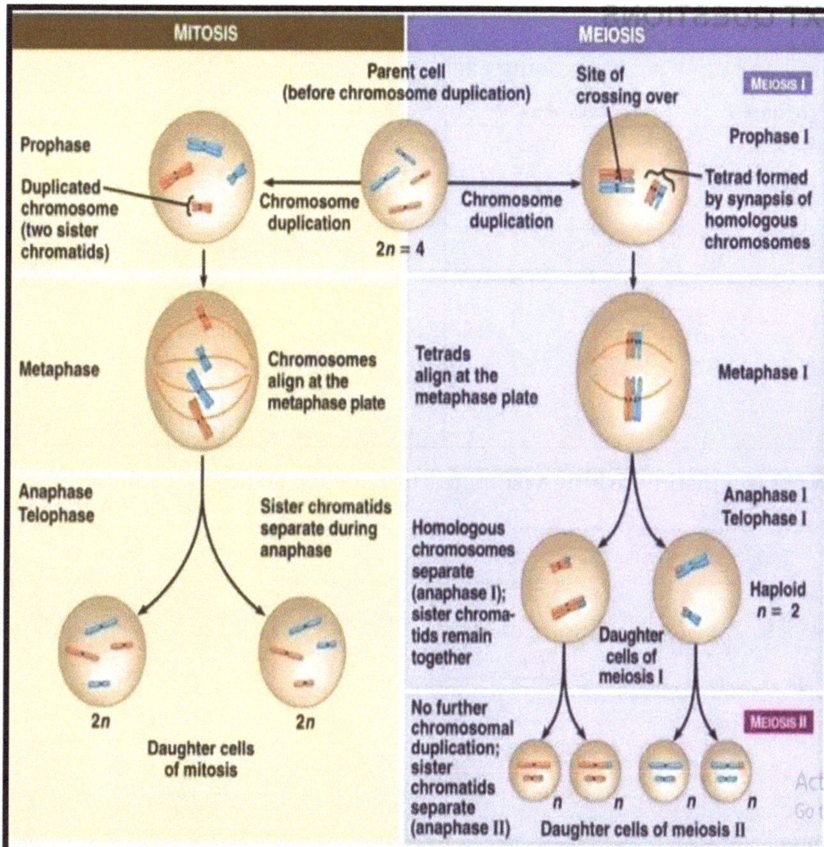

Fig. Diagrammatic representation of difference between mitosis and meiosis

Difference between Meiosis-I and Meiosis-II

S. No.	Meiosis-I	Meiosis-II
1.	Heterotypic division or reductional division.	Homotypic or equational division.
2.	It occurs in dyad stage.	It occurs in tetrad stage.
3.	Homologous chromosomes form metaphase plate.	Separated chromosomes form metaphase plate.
4.	Homologous chromosomes get separated.	Separated chromosomes get divided.
5.	Chromosomes are reduced to half by separation.	Chromosomes are duplicated by division.

INTEXT QUESTIONS

1. Find and draw a cell showing each stage of meiosis.

Prophase I	Metaphase I	Anaphase II	Telophase II

2. What is a distinguishing visible feature of each stage of Prophase I?

Leptotene: ....

....

....

....

....

....

Zygotene: ....

....

....

....

....

....

Pachytene: ....

....

....

....

....

....

Diplotene: ....

Diakinesis: ....

3. What is the significance of meiosis?

4. What is synapsis and crossing over?

5. How can anaphase I and anaphase II be distinguished from each other?

....

....

....

6. Indicate distinguishing feature of metaphase I of meiosis and metaphase of mitosis.

....

....

....

....

....

7. How many daughter cells are produced at the end of meiosis?

....

....

....

....

....

8. The daughter cells produced at the end of meiosis are genetically different. Explain.

....

....

....

....

....

9. Write differences between mitosis and meiosis.

....

....

....

....

....

10. Label each figure with the stage of meiosis that it represents.

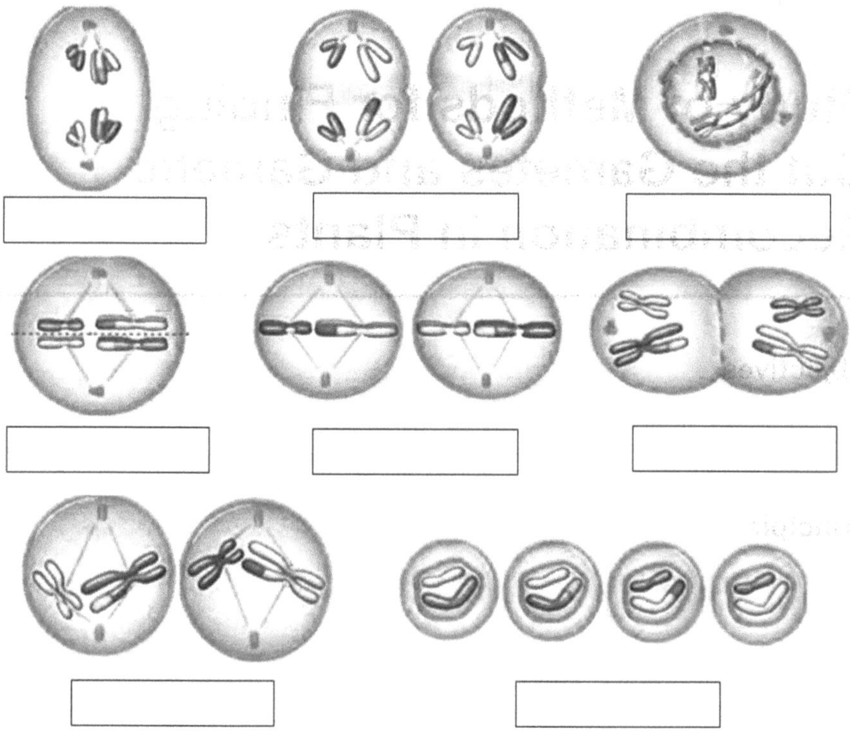

11. Match the following

	Column 1		Column 2
1	Prophase I	**A**	Cytoplasm divide, two daughter cells are formed.
2	Metaphase I	**B**	Homologous chromosome pair up and form tetrad. Crossing over occur
3	Anaphase I	**C**	Homologous chromosomes arrange on equator
4	Telophase I	**D**	Homologous chromosomes moves to opposite poles by shortening of spindle fibres.
5	Cytokinesis I	**E**	Nucleus membrane reforms
6	Metaphase II	**F**	Cytoplasm divide, two daughter cells are formed.
7	Anaphase II	**G**	Chromosomes arrange on equator, not in homologous pair.
8	Cytokinesis II	**H**	Chromatids get separate.

Chapter 6

Study of Methods for Finding Out the Gametes and Gametic Recombination in Plants

Objectives

- Find out the number and types of gametes and gametic recombination in monohybrid, dihybrid and trihybrid crosses.

Principle

Gametes are reproductive cells that join together to form a new cell called a zygote during sexual reproduction. Pollen in seed-bearing plants, is the gametophyte producing male gamete. Female gametes (ovules) are included in the ovary of plant. At maturity a sexually reproducing individuals forms the gametes. Homozygote generate only one form of gamete. Homozygous referring to a diploid cell or organism possessing two identical alleles of a specific gene (e.g. AA or aa). Heterozygote generate different types of gametes. Heterozygous referring to a diploid cell or organism possessing two different alleles of a specific gene (e.g. Aa).

Method of Gamete Formation

1. **Bracket method or Fork line method**: Every allele from one pair of gene is combined with every allele from other pairs which are included in the genotypes
   E.g. AaBb

A < B → AB
A < b → Ab

a < B → aB
a < b → ab

2. **Algebric Method** Both members of every pair of genes from given genotype are written by inserting "+" sign between them

E.g. AaBb

A + a

B + b

AB, aB, Ab, ab

Ques. How many number of gametes will formed from the following genotypes?

(a) Aa

(b) AABb

(c) AaBbCc

Solution.

(a) Aa – A, a   Selfing

(b) AABb

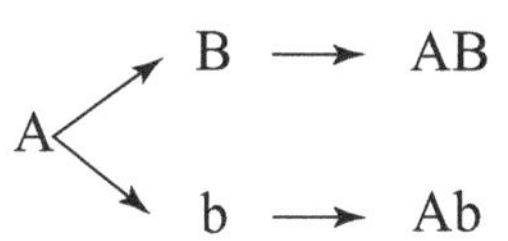

(c) AaBbCc

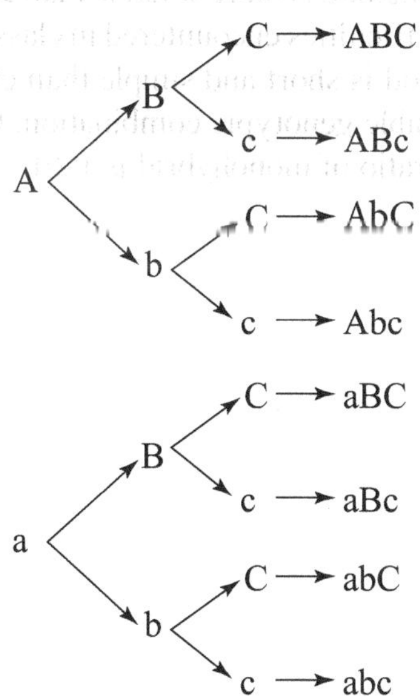

Method of Finding Gametic Recombination

1. Checker Board Method

British Geneticist R. C. Punnet introduced this method. According to this method, male gametes are entered in the first horizontal column and female gametes in the first vertical row. Then female gametes are coupled with every male gamete and genotypic constitutions of zygotes are placed in the checker board.

E.g. **AaBb** **x** **AaBb**

Male Gametes

Female Gametes	AB	Ab	aB	ab
AB	AABB	AABb	AaBB	AaBb
Ab	AABb	AAbb	AaBb	Aabb
aB	AaBB	AaBb	aaBB	aaBb
ab	AaBb	Aabb	aaBb	aabb

2. Bracket Method or Forked Method

This method is similar to bracket method of gamete formation. When more than one genes are considered the bracket method is more suitable than checker board method which is time consuming, difficulties encountered in classifying and chances of error are more. This method is short and simple than checker board and can be used to find out all possible genotypic combination. On the basis of law of segregation the genotypic ratio of monohybrid is 1:2:1.

E.g. AaBb

Aa- Gametic recombination 1AA:2Aa:1aa

Bb- Gametic recombination 1BB:2Bb:1bb

1AA	1BB →	1AABB
	2Bb →	2AABb
	1bb →	1AAbb
2Aa	1BB →	2AaBB
	2Bb →	4AaBb
	1bb →	2Aabb
1aa	1BB →	1aaBB
	2Bb →	2aaBb
	1bb →	1aabb

> ***Note:***
> - Number of different types of gametes produced by an individual is equal to 2^n.
> - Types of zygotes produced by selfing of a genotype is equal to 3^n.
> - Where, 'n' is number of heterozygous gene pair.

Table 1: Possible number of gametes produced from different genotypes

S. No.	Genotype	Number of heterozygous pair (n)	Number of gametes produced (2^n)	Types of possible gametes
1.	AA	0	$2^0 = 1$	A
2.	aa	0	$2^0 = 1$	a
3.	Aa	1	$2^1 = 2$	A, a
4.	AaBb	2	$2^2 = 4$	AB, Ab, aB, ab
5.	AABb	1	$2^1 = 2$	AB, Ab
6.	AaBB	1	$2^1 = 2$	AB, aB
7.	AaBbCc	3	$2^3 = 8$	ABC, ABc, AbC, Abc, aBC, aBc, abC, abc
8.	AaBbCcDd	4	$2^3 = 16$	ABCD, ABCd, ABcD, ABcd, AbCD, AbCd, AbcD, Abcd, aBCD, aBCd, aBcD, aBcd, abCD, abCd, abcD, abcd

Table 2: Possible types of zygotes produced by selfing of genotypes

S. No.	Genotype	Number of heterozygous pair (n)	Number of gametes produced (3n)	Possible types of zygote produced
1.	AA	0	$3^0 = 1$	AA
2.	aa	0	$3^0 = 1$	aa
3.	Aa	1	$3^1 = 3$	AA, Aa. aa
4.	AaBb	2	$3^2 = 9$	AABB, AABb, AAbb, AaBB, AaBb, Aabb, aaBB, aaBb, aabb
5.	AABb	1	$3^1 = 3$	AABB, AABb, AAbb
6.	AaBB	1	$3^1 = 3$	AABB, AaBB, aaBB
7.	AaBbCc	3	$3^3 = 27$	AABBCC, AABBCc, AABBcc, AABbCC, AABbCc, AABbcc, AAbbCC, AAbbCc, AAbbcc, AaBBCC, AaBBCc, AaBBcc, AaBbCC, AaBbCc, AaBbcc, AabbCC, AabbCc, Aabbcc, aaBBCC, aaBBCc, aaBBcc, aaBbCC, aaBbCc, aaBbcc, aabbCC, aabbCc, aabbcc

Shortcut method of finding genetic ratios

We can find out the phenotypic, genotypic and test cross ratios of dihybrid, trihybrid, tetrahybrid, pentahybrid etc. easily by using the genetic ratios of monohybrid cross.

Steps:

1. You should know the phenotypic, genotypic and test cross ratios of monohybrid.
2. Break the given genotype in monohybrid combination. Eg. AaBb i.e., Aa and Bb.
3. Write the genetic ratio of each monohybrid combination as (3:1) × (3:1).
4. Multiply the genetic ratios, to get the result.

Example: Find out the phenotypic, genotypic and test cross ratios of AaBb.

As we know the phenotypic ratio, genotypic ratio and test cross ratio of monohybrid genotype is 3:1, 1:2:1 and 1:1:1:1.

A. Calculation of phenotypic ratio of AaBb

As we know the phenotypic ratio of monohybrid = 3:1

There are two monohybrid combination in genotype AaBb i.e. Aa and Bb

For each monohybrid combination, phenotypic ratio is 3:1

We can write phenotypic ratio of AaBb as (3:1) × (3:1)

Multiply as –

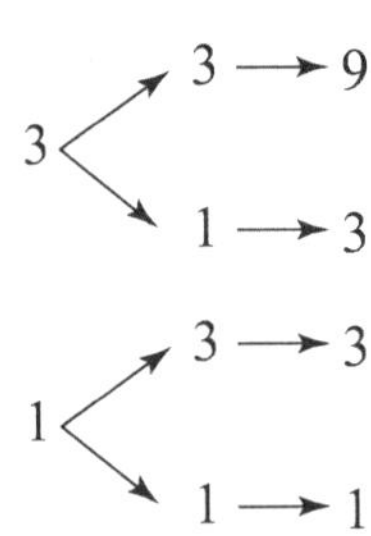

Result: The phenotypic of genotype AaBb is 9:3:3:1

B. Calculation of genotypic ratio of AaBb

As we know the genotypic ratio of monohybrid = 1:2:1

There are two monohybrid combination in genotype AaBb i.e., Aa and Bb

For each monohybrid combination, genotypic ratio is 1:2:1

We can write genotypic ratio of AaBb as (1:2:1) × (1:2:1)

Multiply as:

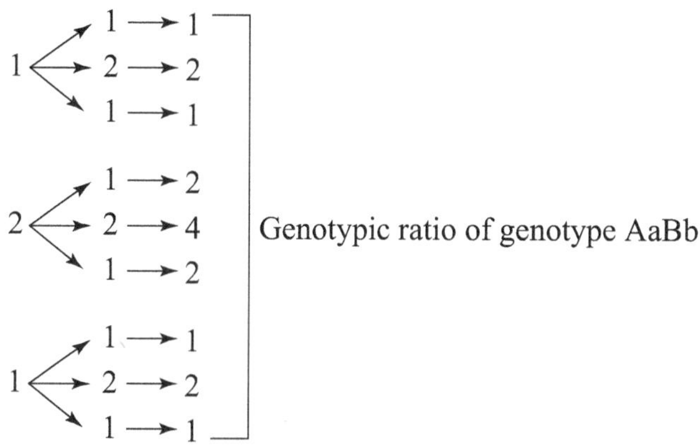

Result: The genotypic of genotype AaBb is 1:2:1:2:4:2:1:2:1

C. Calculation of test cross ratio of AaBb

As we know the test cross ratio of monohybrid = 1:1

There are two monohybrid combination in genotype AaBb i.e. Aa and Bb

For each monohybrid combination, test cross ratio is 1:1

We can write test cross ratio of AaBb as (1:1) × (1:1)

Multiply as:

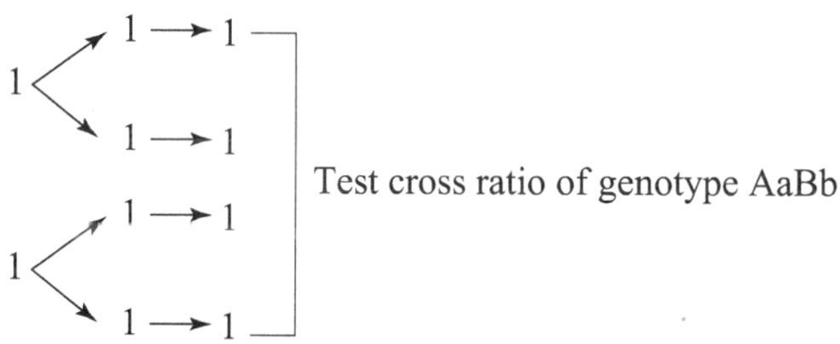

Result: The test cross of genotype AaBb is 1:1:1:1

Table 3: Summary of different genetic ratios calculated using shortcut method

S. No.	Genotype	Number of monohybrid combination	Phenotypic ratio	Genotypic ratio	Test cross ratio
1.	Aa	1	3:1	1:2:1	1:1
2.	AaBb	2 (Aa,Bb)	(3:1) × (3:1) = 9:3:3:1	(1:2:1) × (1:2:1) = 1:2:1:2:4:2:1:2:1	(1:1) × (1:1) = 1:1:1:1
3.	AaBbCc	3 (Aa, Bb, Cc)	(3:1) × (3:1) × (3:1) = 27:9:9:9:3:3:3:1	(1:2:1) × (1:2:1) × (1:2:1) = 1:2:1:2:4:2:1:2:1: 2:4:2:4:8:4:2:4:2: 1:2:1:2:4:2:1:2:1	(1:1) x (1:1) × (1:1) = 1:1:1:1:1:1:1:1
4.	AaBbCcDd	4 (Aa, Bb, Cc, Dd)	(3:1) × (3:1) × (3:1) × (3:1) = 81:27:27:27:9:9:9:3: 27:9:9:9:3:3:3:1	(1:2:1) × (1:2:1) × (1:2:1) × (1:2:1) = 1:2:1:2:4:2:1:2:1:2:4:2 :4:8:4:2:4:2:1:2:1:2:4: 2:1:2:1:2:4:2:4:8:4:2:4 :2:4:8:4:8:16:8:4:8:4:2 :4:2:4:8:4:2:4:2	(1:1) × (1:1) × (1:1) × (1:1) = 1:1:1:1:1:1:1:1: 1:1:1:1:1:1:1:1

INTEXT QUESTIONS

1. Define gamete.

....

....

....

....

....

2. Calculate the possible type of gametes produced from the following genotypes.

(i) AABbCC

....

....

....

....

....

(ii) AaBbCC

....

....

....

....

....

(iii) AaBbCCDd

....

....

....

....

....

(iv) AABBCCDD

....

....

....

....

....

3. A plant of F_1 generation has AABbCc on selfing of this plant. What is the phenotypic ratio in F_2 generation?

....

....

....

....

....

....

4. Total number of offsprings formed by the cross of AABbCc × AaBbCc.

....

....

....

....

....

....

5. When genotype aaBBcc is crossed with AaBbCc. Then the ratio of hybrid for all the three genes is:

....

....

....

....

....

6. In pea plants, purple flowers (P) are dominate white flowers (p) and green pods (G) dominate yellow pods (g). What are the feasible genotypes for a cross between pea plant with genotype PpGG and ppGg? How many squares do you need to analyse this cross in Punnett square?

....

....

....

....

....

....

....

....

....

....

....

....

....

....

....

....

....

....

....

....

....

....

....

7. In garden pea, yellow seed colour (Y) is dominant over green (y) and round seed shape (R) is dominant over wrinkled (r). The two character pairs segregate independently. Determine the genotype of the parents in the crosses: A green wrinkled offspring is obtained from a cross of yellow round x yellow wrinkled. What other offspring may be expected from this cross and in what proportion?

....

....

....

....

....

....

....

....

8. In fowls the dominant genes R (rose comb) and P (pea comb) if present together produces walnut comb. The recessive alleles of both in homozygous condition produce single comb. What will be the comb character of offspring of the following crosses?

   (a) RrPp x RrPp (b) RrPp x rrPp

   (c) RrPp x Rrpp (d) RrPp x rrpp

....

....

....

....

....

....

....

....

....

....

Chapter 7

Study of Monohybrid Cross

Objectives

- Better understand the monohybrid cross.
- Calculation of monohybrid phenotypic, genotypic and testcross ratios.

Principle

Monohybrid cross deals with thc study of inheritance of one pair of contrasting characters. The alleles of contrasting character selected in the monohybrid cross will show exact dominance and recessive relationship. It is also defined as a cross is made between two true-breeding parents differing for a single trait, producing an F_1 generation. These plants are intercrossed to produce an F_2 generation. Monohybrid crosses study led to the Mendel's law of segregation. Monohybrid cross was first produced in pea by Mendel to explain the "law of segregation". When parents with distinct phenotypes are crossed, in F_1 generation, only one type of plants appears phenotypically. However, segregation can be observed in F_2 progeny and the population can be divided into two phenotypes classes. After counting the individuals. It is observed that 75% of them express the dominant phenotype and 25% of them express recessive phenotype.

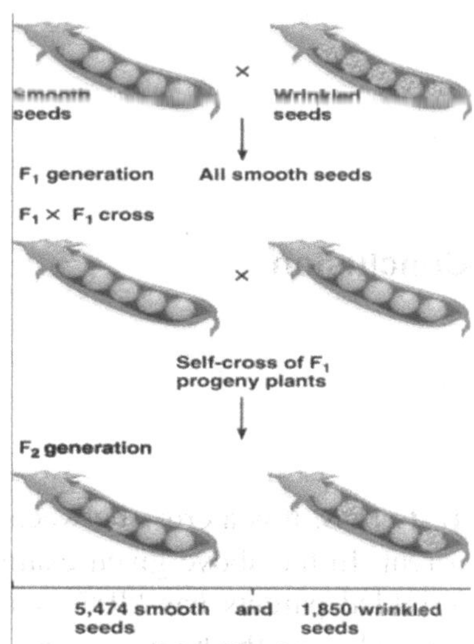

Procedure of monohybrid cross

When a cross was made between one pea parent (P_1) producing round seeds and another parent (P_2) producing wrinkled seeds. In F_1 all seeds were round. This phenomenon by which one trait appears and other does not appear even through factors for both are present is called dominance. When these F_1 grown and selfed, the F_2 progeny showed two type of seeds i.e. round and wrinkled. Study the F_2 progeny and fit into the expected ratio 3:1. The factor for round seed was considered dominant over that for wrinkled which was considered recessive.

Example: In pea plant, Round seed (R) is dominant over the wrinkled seed (r).

Parent - Round seed x Wrinkled seed
RR rr

Gametes ↓ ↓

R r

Fusion ↓

F_1 generation Rr All heterozygous Round seeded (Impure)

↓ Selfing/Self-pollination

F_2 generation Round : Wrinkled
3 : 1 → Phenotypic ratio/Basic ratio

↓

Pure Round : Impure Round : Pure Wrinkled
1 **2** **1** → Genotypic ratio/ Actual ratio

Selfing ↓ Selfing ↓ Selfing ↓

F_3 generation All Round 3 Round : 1 Wrinkled All Wrinkled

Conclusion

F_2 Phenotype : Round and Wrinkled
F_2 Phenotypic ratio : 3 Round: 1 wrinkled
F_2 Genotypes : RR, Rr, rr
F_2 Genotypic ratio : 1 RR: 2 Rr: 1rr

Test cross: It is a cross between a F_1 (hybrid) and the homozygous recessive parent. In the above given example, the F_1 produced by crossing round and wrinkled parents has "Rr" genotype and phenotypically round seeded. In original cross the homozygous recessive parent was wrinkled seeded having "rr" genotypes.

Test cross: F_1 hybrid x Recessive parent

Rr rr

	r
R	Rr (Round)
r	rr (Wrinkled)

Conclusion

Test cross phenotype : Round and Wrinkled

Test cross phenotypic ratio : 1 Round : 1 Wrinkled

Test cross Genotype : Rr, rr

Test cross Genotypic ratio : 1 Rr : 1 rr

Mendel's explanation for his monohybrid cross

- The characters in plants are govern by a pair of contrasting factors. These factors are now known as genes.
- If a plant possess gene for round seed (R), the plant will be round seeded in phenotype. Similarly, if plant possess gene for wrinkled seed (r), the plant will be wrinkle seeded in phenotype.
- In heterozygous condition (Bb), only one allele of a pair is express. One who expressed is known as dominant allele (T), and other whose expression is masked is known as recessive allele (t).
- The alleles will be in pairs in an individual.
- Even though they stay together (like Bb), they never mix each other.
- During gamete formation, both the alleles of a pair (such as Bb) get separated and randomly transferred in to different gametes. Therefore, each gamete contains either 'B' or 'b', is pure for particular trait. This is known as law of segregation or law of purity of gametes.

Problem: In pea plants purple flowers are dominant to white flowers. What will be the phenotype and genotype ratio of off-springs in F_2 generation?

Solution: As per the information given in question:

Purple flowers (P) gene is dominant over white flowers (p) gene.

Pure (homozygous) Purple flower plant = PP

Pure (homozygous) white flower plant = pp

Parent - Purple flower x White flower

PP pp

F_1 generation Pp All heterozygous Round Flower (Impure)

↓ Selfing

F_2 generation Purple : White → Phenotypic ratio

3 : 1

↓

Pure Purple : Impure Purple : Pure White → Genotypic ratio

1 **2** **1**

Conclusion

F_2 Phenotypic ratio : 3 Purple: 1 White

F_2 Genotypic ratio : 1 PP: 2 Pp: 1 pp

Problem: A Tall plant (T) is dominant to dwarf plant (t). If all offspring of a cross are heterozygous, what were the genotypes of the parents?

Solution: If all the off-springs obtained are heterozygous tall, then genotype of one parent will be TT (dominant homozygous) and other parent is tt (recessive homozygous).

Parent- Tall plant x Dwarf plant

TT tt

F_1 generation Tt All heterozygous tall plants (Impure)

Problem: Work out for the genotypes of the parents of the cross between a tall and a dwarf pea plant which result into about one half of the tall and one half of dwarf off-springs.

Solution: Because the off-springs obtained in ratio of 50% tall and 50% dwarf. Therefore, the ratio is 1: 1, so it is a test cross between a pure dwarf (tt) and a heterozygous tall (Tt).

The genotypes may also be shown as follows:

Heterozygous tall (Tt) will form the gametes: T and t.
Pure dwarf (tt) will form the gametes: t and t.

Pure dwarf (tt)	Heterozygous tall (Tt): T	Heterozygous tall (Tt): t
t	Tt Heterozygous tall	tt Pure dwarf
t	Tt Heterozygous tall	tt Pure dwarf

Result: Heterozygous tall = 50% and Pure dwarf = 50%. A ratio of 1:1 will be resulted.

Problem: In case of Mirabilis jalapa, what type of the gametes and flower colours of the off-springs would be produced in the following crosses?

(a) RR x rr (b) Rr xRr

Solution: As we know, flower colour in *Mirabilis jalapa* shows incomplete dominance. Red flowers (R) gene is dominant over white flowers (r) gene. All the F_1 progenies shows pink colour flower due to blending or mixing of characters.

(a) In case of RR x rr

Parent- Red flower RR x White flower rr

F_1 generation Rr Pink flower

Result: All the flowers will be pink colour.

(b) In case of Rr x Rr

Parent - Red flower x Red flower

Rr ↓ Rr ↓

Gametes - R, r R, r

	R	r
R	RR Red	Rr Pink
r	Rr Pink	rr White

Result: A ratio of 1 (Red): 2 (Pink): 1 (White) will be produced.

INTEXT QUESTIONS

Part A: Vocabulary

Match the definitions on the left with the terms on the right.

1.	Genotypes made of the same alleles	A.	Allele
2.	Different forms of genes for a single trait	B.	Dominant
3.	Gene that is always expressed	C.	Heterozygous
4.	Gene that is expressed only in the homozygous state	D.	Homozygous
5.	Genotypes made of two different alleles	E.	Recessive

Part B: Monohybrid Cross Problems

1. Define law of segregation.

....

....

....

....

....

....

....

....

....

2. What will be the appearance of (a) F_1 and (b) F_2 progenies when a pure (homozygous) tall pea plant is crossed with a pure (homozygous) dwarf pea plant?

....

....

....

....

....

....

....

3. When a plant homozygous for tall is crossed with a plant homozygous for dwarf, what will be the appearance of the off-springs of a cross of F_1 with its tall parent?

4. When a plant homozygous for tall is crossed with a plant homozygous for dwarf, what will be the appearance of the off-springs of a cross of F_1 with its dwart parent?

5. In pea, homozygous dominate red flowered plant was crossed with homozygous recessive white flowered plant. Describe the genotype and phenotype of (i) F_1 and F_2 progeny (ii) test cross ratio (iii) Genotypic and phenotypic ratios of F_2.

....

....

....

....

....

....

....

....

....

....

....

....

6. For the following pairs of traits, conduct a monohybrid cross to determine the genotype and phenotype of the offspring.

(a) Dominant trait: A (brown hair)

Recessive trait: a (blonde hair)

Possible Genotypes: ___________

Possible Phenotypes: ___________

	A	a
A		
a		

(b) Dominant trait: B (circular flower)

Recessive trait: b (square flower)

Possible Genotypes: ___________

Possible Phenotypes: ___________

	B	b
b		
b		

7. Explain the inheritance of seed shape in pea plant.

Chapter 8

Study of Dihybrid Cross

Objectives

- Better understand the dihybrid cross.
- Calculation of dihybrid phenotypic, genotypic and testcross ratios.

Principle

A cross is made between two true-breeding parents differing in two pairs of genes, producing an F_1 generation. These plants are inter-crossed to produce an F_2 generation. Mendel second law *i.e.*, Law of independent assortment can be explained by studying the inheritance of two characters at a time, simultaneously. When two phenotypically distinct parents differing with respect to two characters governed by two pair of genes are crossed together. Each pair of genes assorts independently into all possible combination forming four kinds of progeny, two of these are parental type and two are recombinant types.

Procedure

When a cross was made between one pea parent (P_1) producing round seed and yellow cotyledon colour; and another parent (P_2) producing wrinkled seed and green cotyledon colour. In F_1 all seeds were round with yellow cotyledon colour. On selfing of F_1, we get F_2 that produces four phenotypes of seeds i.e., round yellow, round green, wrinkled yellow and wrinkled green in 9:3:3:1 ratio, respectively (phenotypic ratio). This indicates that each gene pair acts independently of the other thereby that the chances for the plant to be round or wrinkled are independent of its chances to be yellow or green.

Example- In pea, one plant producing round seed (R) and yellow cotyledon colour (Y) is dominant over another parent producing the wrinkled seed (r) and green cotyledon colour (y).

Seed form → Round (Dominant)

Seed form → Wrinkled (Recessive)

Cotyledon colour → Yellow (Dominant)
Cotyledon colour → Green (Recessive)

Parent - Round Yellow x Wrinkled Green
RRYY rryy

Gametes
RY ry

Fusion

RrYy

F_1 generation — All Round seed-Yellow colour

Selfing

F_2 generation

Female gametes \ Male gametes	RY	Ry	rY	ry
RY	RRYY	RRYy	RrYY	RrYy
Ry	RRYy	RRyy	RrYy	Rryy
rY	RrYY	RrYy	rrYY	rrYy
ry	RrYy	Rryy	rrYy	rryy

Conclusion

F_2 Phenotype : Round-Yellow, Round-Green, Wrinkled-Yellow, Wrinkled-green

F_2 Phenotypic ratio : 9 Round-Yellow: 3 Round-Green: 3 Wrinkled-Yellow: 1 Wrinkled-green

F_2 Genotypes : RRYY, RrYY, RRYy, RrYy, rrYY, rrYy, RRyy, Rryy, rryy

F_2 Genotypic ratio : 1RRYY: 2RrYY: 2RRYy: 4RrYy: 1rrYY: 2rrYy: 1RRyy: 2Rryy: 1rryy

There are 4 different phenotypes produced i.e. Round yellow, Round green, Wrinkled yellow and Wrinkled green in the 9:3:3:1 ratio, respectively. Out of these four types, two are parental type (Round yellow and Wrinkled green) and two are new combinations (Round green and Wrinkled yellow). There are 9 different genotypes produced which are grouped into 4 genotypic classes viz., R_Y_ (9 individuals), R_yy (3 individuals), rrY_ (3 individuals) and rryy (one individual). These four genotypic classes represent four phenotype i.e., round yellow, round green, wrinkled yellow and wrinkled green.

Test cross: It is a cross between a F_1 (hybrid) and the homozygous recessive parent. In the above given example, the F_1 produced by crossing round-yellow and wrinkled-green parents has "RrYy" genotype and phenotypically round-yellow seeded. In original cross the homozygous recessive parent was wrinkled-green seeded having "rryy" genotype.

Test cross : F_1 hybrid x Recessive parent

RrYy rryy

↓

	ry
RY	RrYy (Round Yellow)
Ry	Rryy (Round Green)
rY	rrYy (Wrinkled Yellow)
ry	rryy (Wrinkled Green)

Conclusion

Test cross phenotype : Round-Yellow, Round-Green, Wrinkled-Yellow, Wrinkled-Green

Test cross phenotypic ratio : 1Round-Yellow: 1Round-Green:1Wrinkled-Yellow:1Wrinkled-Green

Test cross Genotype : RrYy, Rryy, rrYy, rryy

Test cross Genotypic ratio : 1 RrYy: 1 Rryy: 1 rrYy: 1 rryy

Problem: When round and yellow seeded pea plants (YYRR) are crossed with green wrinkled (yyrr) seeded pea plants the F_1 are yellow and round seeded plants (YyRr). What will be the results when this F_1 is crossed with round and yellow seeded parents?

Solution: Following results may be obtained when F_1 (YyRr) are crossed with pure yellow and round seeded parent (YYRR).

Parent - YyRr YYRR

↓ ↓

Gametes- YR, Yr, yR, yr YR

	YR	Yr	yR	yr
YR	YYRR Yellow and round seeded	YYRr Yellow and round seeded	YyRR Yellow and round seeded	YyRr Yellow and round seeded

Result: All the plants will be yellow and round seeded.

Problem: When round and yellow seeded pea plants (YYRR) are crossed with green and wrinkled (yyrr) seeded pea plants the F_1 are yellow and round seeded plants (YyRr). What will be the results when this F_1 is crossed with green and wrinkled seeded (yyrr) parents?

Solution: Following results will be obtained when F_1 (YyRr) are crossed with green and wrinkled seeded (yyrr) parents:

Parent - YyRr yyrr

↓ ↓

Gametes- YR, Yr, yR, yr yr

	YR	Yr	yR	yr
yr	YyRr Yellow and round seeded	Yyrr Yellow and wrinkle seeded	yyRr Green and round seeded	yyrr Green and wrinkle seeded
Ratio:	1	1	1	1

Result: Four different kinds of plants are obtained in 1:1:1:1 ratio.

Problem: Find out the phenotypic value of the offspring of the following cross, in which the genotypes of the parents are given: YYRr x YyRr

Solution:

Parent - YYRr YyRr

Gametes- YR, Yr YR, Yr, yR, yr

	YR	Yr	yR	yr
YR	YYRR Yellow and round seeded	YYRr Yellow and round seeded	YyRR Yellow and round seeded	YyRr Yellow and round seeded
Yr	YYRr Yellow and round seeded	YYrr Yellow and wrinkle seeded	YyRr Yellow and round seeded	Yyrr Yellow and wrinkle seeded

Result: A ratio of 6 (Yellow and round seeded):2 (Yellow and wrinkle seeded) would be resulted.

Difference between monohybrid cross and dihybrid cross

Monohybrid cross	Dihybrid cross
A monohybrid cross is a genetic cross between homozygous individuals with different alleles for a single gene locus.	A monohybrid cross is a genetic cross between individuals with different alleles for two gene loci.
One character is considered and studied.	Two independent characters are considered and studied.
A single pair of gene is involved.	Two pairs of genes are involved.
Predicted phenotypic ratio is 3:1	Predicted phenotypic ratio is 9:3:3:1
Predicted genotypic ratio is 1:2:1	Predicted genotypic ratio is 1:2:1:2:4:2:1:2:1
Predicted test cross ratio is 1:1	Predicted test cross ratio is 1:1:1:1
Important for determining the dominance relationship between the alleles.	Important for assessing the independent assortment of alleles.

INTEXT QUESTIONS

1. In garden peas, tall plant (T) is dominant over dwarf plant (t) and yellow seed (Y) is dominant over green seed (y). How would you find out the genotypes of the following phenotypes?

   (a) Tall plant and green seed (b) Dwarf plant and yellow seeds.

   Also find out the genotypic and phenotype ratio of F_2 population and test cross progeny.

....

....

....

....

....

....

....

....

....

....

....

....

....

....

....

....

....

....

....

....

....

2. In guinea pigs, rough coat is dominant over smooth coat and black coat is dominant over white. Genes for these two characters are located in two different chromosomes. A homozygous rough, black animal is mated with a smooth, white one. Give the genotypes and phenotypes of F_1, gametes produced by F_2 and the genotypes and phenotypes obtained in F_2 and Test cross progenies.

....

....

....

....

....

....

....

....

....

....

....

....

....

....

....

....

....

....

....

....

....

....

....

3. A round seeded plant (R) is dominant to a wrinkled seeded plant (r). What parental genotypes will produce offspring that are 50% homozygous dominant and 50% heterozygous?

....

....

....

....

....

....

....

....

....

....

....

4. A homozygous round seeded plant is crossed with a homozygous wrinkled seeded plant. What percentage of the offspring will also be homozygous?.

....

....

....

....

....

....

....

....

....

....

....

Chapter 9

Working Out Problems Related to Independent Assortment

Objectives

- Better understand the law of independent assortment.

History

The law was proposed by Gregor Johann Mendel with the other laws together called as 'Mendelian laws of inheritance', in 1866. He used pea plant as a model organism, and studied 7 characters.

Principle

The Law of Independent Assortment, also known as "Inheritance Law", states that alleles of different genes assort independently of one another during gamete formation. Independent assortment for two genes can be explained by assuming that the two genes are located in two different chromosomes. The two alleles of a gene will be located in the two homologues of the concerned chromosome. Independent separation of these two pairs of chromosomes at anaphase I of meiosis will lead to the independent segregation of the genes located in them. Thus any allele of one gene is equally likely to combine with any allele of the other gene and pass into the same gamete. Independent segregation of two genes produces four different types of gametes in equal proportion. A random union among these gametes gives rise to sixteen possible zygotes. These zygotes yield a 9:3:3:1 phenotypic ratio, which is known as the typical dihybrid ratio. When two pairs of independent alleles enter into F_1 combination, both of them have their independent dominant effect. These alleles segregate when gametes are formed but the assortment occurs independently at random and quite freely.

Explanation

The cross was made between plants having yellow and round cotyledons and plants having green and wrinkled cotyledons. The F_1 hybrids all had yellow and round seeds. When these F_1 plants were self-fertilized they produced four types of plants in the following proportion:

i. Round and yellow : 9
ii. Wrinkled and yellow : 3
iii. Round and green : 3
iv. Wrinkled and green : 1

Meaning of word assortment is 'random or freely'. Thus probability theorem is applicable to the dihybrid cross experiment. According to basic principle of probability, "Probability of two independent events occurring simultaneously is a product of their individual probabilities". The above results indicate that yellow and green seeds appear in the ratio of 9 + 3:3 + 1 = 3 : 1. Similarly, the round and wrinkled seeds appear in the ratio of 9 + 3:3 + 1 = 12 : 4 or 3:1. The probability of first trait is 3:1, while that of second trait is also 3:1. Thus the dihybrid ratio should be (3:1) × (3:1) = 3 × 3 : 3 × 1 : 1 × 3 : 1 × 1 = 9:3:3:1. This indicates that each of the two pairs of alternative characters viz. yellow-green cotyledon colour is inherited independent of the round-wrinkled character of the cotyledons. It means at the time of gamete formation the factor for yellow colour enters the gametes independent of R or r, i.e., gene Y can be passed on to the gametes either with gene R or r.

Cytological explanation of the results

In the above experiment yellow and round characters are dominant over green and wrinkled characters which can be represented as follows:

i Gene for yellow colour of cotyledons : Y
ii Gene for green colour of cotyledons : y
iii Gene for round character of cotyledons : R
iv Gene for wrinkled character of cotyledons : r

Therefore, plants with yellow and round cotyledons will have their genotype YYRR and those with green and wrinkled cotyledons will have a genotype yyrr. These plants will produce gametes with gene YR and yr respectively. When these plants are cross pollinated, the union of these gametes will produce F_1 hybrids with YyRr genes. When these produce gametes all the four genes have full freedom to assort independently and, therefore, there are possibilities of four combinations in both male and female gametes.

(i) RY (ii) Ry (iii) rY (iv) ry

This shows an excellent example of independent assortment. These gametes can unite at random producing in all 16 different combinations of genes, but presenting four phenotypes in the ratio of 9:3:3:1. Out of 16 possible combinations, 9 are combinations having the alleles for both the traits as dominant, 3 each for 1 allele for a trait dominant & the other allele for other trait as recessive (2 possible combinations, total 6 out of 16), 1 combination where alleles for both the traits are recessive. This agrees with the law of dominance. Now to explain the independent assortment of traits in the progeny of F_2 generation refers the previous chapter.

Problem: In pea plant, yellow cotyledon colour (Y) is dominant to green cotyledon colour (y), and round seed (R) is dominant to wrinkled seed (r). The cotyledon colour gene and the seed form gene are on different chromosomes, so they assort independently, and are not sex linked. In a cross between two RrYy parents, predict the fraction of offspring with round seed and yellow cotyledon colour.

Solution: Following results may be obtained when (RrYy) are crossed with another (RrYy).

Parent - RrYy RrYy

↓ ↓

Gametes – RY, Ry, rY, ry RY, Ry, rY, ry

	RY	Ry	rY	ry
RY	RRYY Round-yellow	RRYy Round-yellow	RrYY Round-yellow	RrYy Round-yellow
Ry	RRYy Round-yellow	RRyy Round-green	RrYy Round-yellow	Rryy Round-green
rY	RrYY Round-yellow	RrYy Round-yellow	rrYY Wrinkle-yellow	rrYy Wrinkle-yellow
ry	RrYy Round-yellow	Rryy Round-green	rrYy Wrinkle-yellow	rryy Wrinkle-green

Result: The probability of obtaining round seed with yellow cotyledon colour = 9/16*100 = 56.25%

INTEXT QUESTIONS

1. Define law of Independent assortment.

....

....

....

....

....

....

....

....

....

....

2. Suppose you cross a pure-breeding, black-coated dog with curly fur to a pure-breeding, yellow-coated dog with straight fur. In the F_1 generation, all the puppies have straight, black coats. Next, you interbreed the F_1 dogs with one another to get an F_2 generation.

   If coat colour and coat texture are controlled by two genes that assort independently, what fraction of the F_2 puppies are expected to have yellow, straight fur?

....

....

....

....

....

....

....

....

....

....

Chapter 10

Working Out Problems Related to Chi-square (χ^2) Test

Objectives

- Chi-square test for goodness of fit of genetic ratios.

Introduction

Karl Pearson developed the chi square test of statistical significance which is commonly used in Mendelian and population genetics. Chi square (χ^2) test is a test of statistical significance which is used to test the significance difference between observed and expected frequencies or ratios. The purpose of χ^2 test is to decide if a set of observed data is according to an expected ratio or if it agrees well with an expected or theoretical distribution.

The chi square test of independence allow us to evaluate whether the segregation of alleles at one locus is independent of the segregation of alleles at another locus. To distinguish between inheritance patterns that obey Mendel's laws versus those that do not, a conventional strategy is to make crosses and then quantitatively analyze the offspring's. Based on the observed outcome, an experimenter may make a tentative hypothesis. For example, it may seem that the data are obeying Mendel's laws. Hypothesis testing provides an objective, statistical method to evaluate whether the observed data really agree with the hypothesis.

The underlying principles behind a statistical approach is to evaluate the goodness of fit between the observed data and the data that are predicted from a hypothesis. This is sometimes called a null hypothesis because it assumes there is no real difference between the observed and expected values. A high deviation would be found between the observed and expected values. If this occurs, the hypothesis is rejected. Hopefully, the experimenter can subsequently propose an alternative hypothesis that has a better fit with the data.

The null hypothesis is a particular claim concerning how the data is distributed. More will be said about the construction of the null hypothesis later. The null and alternative hypotheses for each chi square test can be stated as

$$H_0: O_1 = E_1$$
$$H_1: O_i \neq E_i$$

If the claim made in the null hypothesis is true, the observed and the expected values are close to each other and $O_i - E_i$ is small for each category. When the observed data does not conform to what has been expected on the basis of the null hypothesis, the difference between the observed and expected values, $O_i - E_i$, is large. The chi square statistic is thus small when the null hypothesis is true, and large when the null hypothesis is not true. Exactly how large the χ^2 value must be in order to be considered large enough to reject the null hypothesis, can be determined from the level of significance and the chi square table.

The chi square test is based on the difference between the observed and the expected values for each category. The general formula for calculating χ^2 may be written as

$$\chi^2 = \sum \frac{(0 - E)^2}{E}$$

Where,

$\sum$ refers to summation,

O is the observed frequency,

E is the expected frequency.

Degree of freedom: The degree of freedom (*df*) is one less than the total number of classes in the data.

$$df = (n - 1)$$

The reason why it is important to consider degrees of freedom is that the value of the chi-square statistic is calculated as the sum of the squared deviations for all of the possible categories. The more categories considered increases the chance for random error; therefore, the critical value for chi-square must increase as the degrees of freedom increase.

Requirement for χ^2 test

1. Quantitative data.
2. One or more categories.
3. Independent observations.
4. Adequate sample size (at least 10).
5. Simple random sample.
6. Data in frequency form.
7. All observations must be used.

Procedure

Propose a hypothesis that allow us to calculate the expected values based on Mendel's law. Computation of chi-square from the observed data required observed frequencies, expected frequencies (according to Mendelian 3:1 or

9:3:3:1 ratios) for each of the class, calculate deviation of observed frequency from the expected one for each of the class. The + and – signs of the deviations are removed by squaring the deviations. Now the deviation squares are divided by the expected frequencies of the respective classes. The summation for all quotients obtained give the calculated value of chi-square.

Concluding the calculated chi-square value

The value of χ^2 at 5% level of significance or 0.05 probability against the appropriate degree of freedom (df) is obtained from the χ^2 table.

If the calculated χ^2 value < table χ^2 value at $n - 1$ df at 0.05 probability, the results are non-significant. This indicate that the null hypothesis is accepted. The deviation of observed data from the expected frequencies is accepted to be purely due to chance. Therefore, it is concluded that the observed data are in accordance with the expected ratio (3:1 or 9:3:3:1).

If the calculated χ^2 value ≥ table χ^2 value at n – 1 df at 0.05 probability, the results are significant. This indicate that the null hypothesis is rejected. Therefore, it is concluded that the observed data are not according to the expected ratio (3:1 or 9:3:3:1).

Example 1: In the garden pea, yellow cotyledon colour is dominant to green, and inflated pod shape is dominant to the constricted form. Considering both of these traits jointly in self-fertilized dihybrids, the progeny appeared in the following numbers:

193	green, inflated
184	yellow constricted
556	yellow, inflated
61	green, constricted

Do these genes assort independently? Support your answer using Chi-square analysis.

Solution: Genes assort independently (are NOT on the same chromosome and NOT linked) if they follow the 9:3:3:1 rule resulting from a dihybrid cross. In this dihybrid cross:

Yellow Cotyledons- Inflated pod YYPP	x	Green cotyledons- Constricted form yypp

F_1 generation: All offspring's have Yellow Cotyledons-Inflated pod

YyPp

↓ Selfing

F_2 generation: Obtained four class (Total = 994)

556 yellow, inflated
184 yellow constricted
193 green, inflated
61 green, constricted

Step 1: Propose a hypothesis that allow us to calculate the expected values based on Mendel's law.

$$H_0: O_i = E_i$$
$$H_1: O_i \neq E_i$$

Step 2: The total observed value is 994, so I found the expected values as so:

9/16 * 994 = 559 yellow, inflated
3/16 * 994 = 186 yellow constricted
3/16 * 994 = 186 green, inflated
1/16 * 994 = 62 green, constricted

Step 3: Now calculate the chi-square value by use of observed and expected value as

Phenotype	Observed value (O)	Expected value (E)	O-E	$(O-E)^2$	$(O-E)^2/E$
yellow, inflated	556	559	–3	9	0.016
yellow constricted	184	186	–2	4	0.02
green, inflated	193	186	7	49	0.26
green, constricted	61	62	–1	1	0.02

Now, compare the calculated χ^2 value with table χ^2 value at $(n - 1)$ d.f. at 5% level of significance, to make conclusion regarding the validity of null hypothesis:

Calculated χ^2 value = 0.316

Table χ^2 value at 3 d.f. at 5% level of significance = 7.815

Calculated value is much lower than the tabulated value, so we cannot reject the null hypothesis. The genes assort independently according to a 9:3:3:1 ratio.

Example 2: In a cross between green fruited and white fruited eggplant the F_1s produced mosaic green coloured fruits. In F_2, out of 45 plants studied 12 green, 24 mosaic green and 9 white fruited were observed. Test the goodness of fit. What are the genotypes of parents and offspring?

Assumption: Fruit colour is governed by one pair of gene showing incomplete dominance and segregation taking place in the ratio of 1:2:1.

Solution: Green fruit colour (G) is incompletely dominant over white (g) and F_1 produces mosaic green fruits. In the F_2, segregation took place in ratio of 1:2:1. In this cross:

Green fruit x White fruit
GG gg

F_1 generation: All offspring's have green mosaic fruit
Gg

↓ Selfing

Obtained three class (Total = 45)

F_2 generation: 12 Green
24 Mosaic green
09 White

Step 1: Propose a hypothesis that allow us to calculate the expected values.

$$H_0: O_i = E_i$$
$$H_1: O_i \neq E_i$$

Step 2: The total observed value is 45, so we found the expected values as so:

1/4 * 45 = 11.25 Green
2/4 * 45 = 22.50 Mosaic green
1/4 * 45 = 11.25 White

Step 3: Now calculate the chi-square value by use of observed and expected value as

Phenotype	Observed value (O)	Expected value (E)	O-E	$(O-E)^2$	$(O-E)^2/E$
Green	12	11.25	+0.75	9	0.050
Mosaic green	24	22.50	+1.5	4	0.100
White	09	11.25	–2.25	49	0.450
Total	45				0.600

Now, compare the calculated χ^2 value with table χ^2 value at (n-1) d.f. at 5% level of significance, to make conclusion regarding the validity of null hypothesis:

Calculated χ^2 value = 0.600

Table χ^2 value at 2 d.f. at 5% level of significance = 5.99

Calculated χ^2 value is much lower than the tabulated value, so we cannot reject the null hypothesis. The deviation between observed and expected values are not significant. The fit is good for assumed ratio 1:2:1.

Table 1. Critical value of the chi-square (χ^2) distribution.

d.f.	.995	.99	.975	.95	9	.1	.05	.025	.01
1	0.00	0.00	0.00	0.00	0.02	2.71	3.84	5.02	6.63
2	0.01	0.02	0.05	0.10	0.21	4.61	5.99	7.38	9.21
3	0.07	0.11	0.22	0.35	0.58	6.25	7.81	9.35	11.34
4	0.21	0.30	0.48	0.71	1.06	7.78	9.49	11.14	13.28
5	0.41	0.55	0.83	1.15	1.61	9.24	11.07	12.83	15.09
6	0.68	0.87	1.24	1.64	2.20	10.64	12.59	14.45	16.81
7	0.99	1.24	1.69	2.17	2.83	12.02	14.07	16.01	18.48
8	1.34	1.65	2.18	2.73	3.49	13.36	15.51	20.48	23.21
9	1.73	2.09	2.70	3.33	4.17	14.68	16.92	19.02	21.67
10	2.16	2.56	3.25	3.94	4.87	15.99	18.31	20.48	23.21
11	2.60	3.05	3.82	4.57	5.58	17.28	19.68	21.92	24.72
12	3.07	3.57	4.40	5.23	6.30	18.55	21.03	23.34	26.22
13	3.57	4.11	5.01	5.89	7.04	19.81	22.36	24.74	27.69
14	4.07	4.66	5.63	6.57	7.79	21.06	23.68	26.12	29.14
15	4.60	5.23	6.26	7.26	8.55	22.31	25.00	27.19	30.58
16	5.14	5.81	6.91	7.96	9.31	23.54	26.30	28.85	32.00
17	5.70	6.41	7.56	8.67	10.09	24.77	27.59	30.19	33.41
18	6.26	7.01	8.23	9.39	10.86	25.99	25.87	31.53	34.81
19	6.84	7.63	8.91	10.12	11.65	27.20	30.14	32.85	36.19
20	7.43	8.26	9.59	10.85	12.44	28.41	31.41	34.17	37.57
22	8.64	9.54	10.98	12.34	14.04	30.81	33.92	36.78	40.29
24	9.89	10.86	12.10	13.85	15.66	33.20	36.42	39.36	42.98
26	11.16	12.20	13.84	15.38	17.29	35.56	38.89	41.92	45.64
28	12.46	16.56	15.31	16.69	18.94	37.92	41.34	44.46	48.28
30	13.79	14.95	16.79	18.49	20.60	40.26	43.77	46.98	50.89
32	15.13	16.36	18.29	20.07	22.27	42.58	46.19	19.48	53.49
34	16.50	17.79	19.81	21.66	23.95	44.90	48.60	51.97	56.06
38	19.29	20.69	22.88	24.88	27.34	49.51	53.38	56.90	61.16
42	22.14	23.65	26.00	28.14	30.77	54.09	28.12	61.75	66.21
46	25.04	20.66	29.16	31.44	34.22	58.64	62.83	66.62	71.20
50	27.99	29.71	32.36	34.76	37.69	63.17	67.50	71.42	76.15
55	31.73	33.57	36.40	38.96	42.06	68.80	73.31	77.38	82.29
60	35.53	34.78	40.48	43.19	46.46	74.40	79.08	83.30	88.38
65	39.38	41.44	44.60	47.45	50.88	79.97	84.82	89.18	94.42
70	43.28	45.44	48.76	51.74	55.33	85.83	90.53	65.02	100.43
75	47.21	49.48	52.94	56.05	59.79	91.06	96.22	100.84	106.39
80	51.17	53.54	57.15	60.39	64.28	96.58	101.88	106.63	112.33
85	55.17	57.63	61.39	64.75	68.78	102.08	107.52	112.39	118.24
90	59.20	61.75	65.65	69.13	73.29	107.57	113.15	118.14	124.12
95	63.25	65.90	69.92	73.52	77.82	113.04	118.75	123.86	129.97
100	67.33	70.06	74.22	77.93	82.36	118.50	121.34	129.56	135.81

INTEXT QUESTIONS

1. In maize, starchy grain trait is dominant to sugary grain trait and red seed grain colour is dominant to white. In F_2 generation of a cross between starchy red and sugary white, 400 seeds were obtained in the following classes: Starchy red = 180, starchy white 100, sugary red = 110 and sugary white = 10. Test the data for independent assortment.

....

....

....

....

....

....

....

....

....

....

....

....

....

....

....

....

....

....

....

....

....

....

2. In a dihybrid cross between two varieties, the following segregation was observed in the F_2 generation A-B = 289, A-bb = 92, aaB = 73 aabb = 26. Test if two genes are segregating independently or not.

....

....

....

....

....

....

....

....

....

....

....

....

....

....

....

....

....

....

....

....

....

....

....

....

....

3. A cross between orange cotyledon coloured strain of lentil with yellow cotyledon resulted in F_1 which produced orange coloured cotyledons. Study of F_2 seeds showed 586 orange cotyledon and yellow cotyledon. Test the data using chi-square test. Explain the result genetically. (Assumption: The character cotyledon colour is governed by one pair of gene and segregation is taking place into the ratio of 3:1).

....

....

....

....

....

....

....

....

....

....

....

....

....

....

....

....

....

....

....

....

....

....

....

Chapter 11

Working Out Problems Related to Linkage

Objectives

- Detection of linkage using Chi-square test for goodness of fit.

Introduction

The tendency of two or more genes to stay together during inheritance is known as linkage and it is the consequence of the concerned genes being located in the same chromosome. Linked genes do not show independent segregation, as a result the ratios obtained in F_2 and test cross generation are significantly different from the expected ratios of 9:3:3:1 and 1:1:1:1, respectively.

Detection of linkage χ^2 using test

In genetic experiments, when the material under study is segregating simultaneously for two characters, it may be of interest to know whether the two characters are inherited independently or they are linked. The χ^2 test can be used for this purpose. χ^2 test is used in detecting linkage in back crosses and inter crosses.

First the χ^2 is computed based on the theoretical segregating ratios. If χ^2 is not significant it may be concluded that the loci segregate independently. If χ^2 is significant we may suspect linkage between the loci. The χ^2 is then partitioned into components assignable to different factors.

(a) Detection of linkage from Inter-crosses

In F_2 progeny, each of the two gene pair (A/a and B/b) individually segregate in 3:1 ratio, simultaneously, segregation of these two gene pairs expected to be in the phenotypic ratio of 9:3:3:1 (A_B_, A_bb, aaB_ and aabb). If the segregation for genes A/a and B/b separately yield 3:1 ratio and the chi-square (χ^2) for independence of segregation for genes A/a and B/b are not segregating independently (not in 9:3:3:1) i.e. they are linked.

Table 1. Detection of linkage from inter cross AaBb × AaBb.

Phenotypic Classes	A_B_	A_bb	aaB_	aabb
Observed frequency	f_1	f_2	f_3	f_4
Probability	9/16	3/16	3/16	1/16

$$\chi^2_A = [(f_1 + f_2) - 3(f_3 + f_4)]^2/3n$$

Similarly, we obtain

$$\chi^2_B = [(f_1 + f_3) - 3(f_2 + f_4)]^2/3n$$

$$\chi^2_L = [(f_1 + 9f_4) - 3(f_2 + f_3)]^2/9n$$

Each χ^2 has 1 d.f.

Conclusion

If the χ^2 test for inter cross AaBb × AaBb is significant (χ^2 cal. > χ^2 tab.), the observed frequencies of phenotypic classes 'A_ and aa' and 'B_and bb' are in the 3:1 ratio (χ^2cal.< χ^2 tab) and the χ^2 test for independence of segregation of genes A/a and B/b is significant (χ^2 cal.> χ^2 tab) indicating that genes A/a and B/b are not segregating independently, i.e., are linked.

(b) Detection of linkage from back crosses (Test cross)

The back cross AaBb × aabb will produce the phenotype AaBb, Aabb, aaBb and aabb in the ratio 1:1:1:1, if there is no linkage. In an experiment the frequency of the phenotypes may be observed as f_1, f_2, f_3 and f_4, respectively. Based on the expected ratio, we can compute the expected frequency and χ^2. If the χ^2 is significant we use the contrast 'A versus a' and 'B versus b' to test whether the segregation ratio 1:1 at each locus is disturbed or not. The contrast (AaBb + aabb) versus (Aabb + aaBb) is used to detect the linkage, and it is termed as linkage.

Table 2. Detection of linkage from back cross AaBb × aabb.

Phenotypic Classes	AaBb	Aabb	aaBb	aabb
Observed frequency	f_1	f_2	f_3	f_4
Probability	1/4	1/4	1/4	1/4

Using this table we can compute the χ^2 value for three contrasts

$$\chi^2_A = [(f_1 + f_2) - (f_3 + f_4)]^2/n$$

$$\chi^2_B = [(f_1 + f_3) - (f_2 + f_4)]^2/n$$

Similarly,

$$\chi^2_L = [(f_1 + f_4) - (f_2 + f_3)]^2/n$$

which is the test statistic for the detection of linkage. Each χ^2 has 1 d.f.

Conclusion

If the χ^2 test for back cross AaBb × aabb is significant (χ^2 cal. > χ^2 tab.), the observed frequencies of phenotypic classes 'A_ and aa' and 'B_and bb' are in the 3:1 ratio (χ^2 cal.< χ^2 tab) and the χ^2 test for independence of segregation of genes A/a and B/b is significant (χ^2 cal.> χ^2 tab) indicating that genes A/a and B/b are not segregating independently, i.e. are linked.

Linkage relationships

Linkage relationships from a two-point test cross: The parental combinations will tend to stay together in the majority of the progeny and the recombinant types will always be the least frequent classes. From this information, the mode of linkage (coupling-repulsion) may be determined for the dihybrid parent.

Parent:	Dihybrid Parent	×	Testcross Parent
	Aa/Bb	↓	b/ab
	(Linkage relationship unknown)		

F_1:			
	AaBb	42%	Parental type
	aabb	42%	Parental type
	Aabb	8%	Recombinant types
	aaBb	8%	Recombinant types

The test cross parent contribute 'ab' to each progeny. The remaining genes come from the dihybrid parent. Thus A and B must have on one chromosome of dihybrid parent and 'a' and 'b' on the other i.e., in coupling phase (AB/ab) because, these were the combinations that appeared with greatest frequency in the progeny.

Parent:	Dihybrid Parent	x	Testcross Parent
	Aa/Bb	↓	ab/ab
	(Linkage relationship unknown)		

F_1:			
	AaBb	8%	Recombinant types
	aabb	8%	Recombinant types
	Aabb	42%	Parental types
	aaBb	42%	Parental types

The testcross parent contribute "ab" to each progeny. The remaining genes come from the dihybrid parent. Thus "A" and "b" must have been on one chromosome of dihybrid parent "a" and "B" on the other i.e. in repulsion phase (Ab/aB) because these were the combination that appeared with greatest frequency in the progeny.

The tendency of genes to recombine is equally strong whether they are in coupling or repulsion phase.

Example: For the inter cross AaBb × AaBb, the phenotype in F_2 sample are classified as follows

A_B_ = 96, A_bb = 16, aaB_ = 18 aabb = 30 Total = 160

They are expected to occur in a 9:3:3:1 ratio. Test whether the two loci A and B are linked.

Solution: The total observed value is 160, so I found the expected values as so:

9/16 * 160 = 90 A_B_
3/16 * 160 = 30 A_bb
3/16 * 160 = 30 aaB_
1/16 * 160 = 10 aabb

Detection of linkage from inter cross AaBb × AaBb.

Phenotypic Classes	A_B_	A_bb	aaB_	aabb
Observed frequency (O)	96	16	18	30
Expected frequency (E)	90	30	30	10
(O-E)	+6	-14	-12	+20
$(O-E)^2$	36	196	144	400
$(O-E)^2/E$	0.40	6.53	4.8	40

Now, compare the calculated χ^2 value with table χ^2 value at $(n-1)$ d.f. at 5% level of significance, to make conclusion regarding the validity of 9:3:3:1.

Calculated χ^2 value = 51.73

Table χ^2 value at 3 d.f. at 5% level of significance – 7.815

Calculated value is much higher than the tabulated value, so the χ^2 is significant. We can reject the null hypothesis. The genes cannot assort independently according to a 9:3:3:1 ratio.

$$\chi^2_A = [(f_1 + f_2) - 3(f_3 + f_4)]^2 / 3n$$
$$= [(96+16) - 3(18+30)]^2 / 3(160)$$
$$= 2.13$$

$$\chi^2_B = [(f_1 + f_3) - 3(f_2 + f_4)]^2 / 3n$$
$$= [(96 + 18) - 3(16 + 30)]^2 / 3(160)$$
$$= 1.20$$

$$\chi^2_L = [(f_1 + 9f_4) - 3(f_2 + f_3)]^2 / 9n$$
$$= [96 + 9(30) - 3(16 + 18)]^2 / 9\ (160)$$
$$= (366 - 102)^2 / 1440$$

$= 69696 / 1440$
$= 48.40$

Each χ^2 has 1 d.f.

Table χ^2 value at 1 d.f. at 5% level of significance = 3.841

Table χ^2 value at 1 d.f. at 1% level of significance = 6.635

Note that $\chi^2_A + \chi^2_B + \chi^2_L = \chi^2$

Here, χ^2_A and χ^2_B are not significant at 5% and 1% level of significance, we conclude that the two loci A and B are linked.

Point to be remember

A. Difference between linkage and crossing over

	Linkage	Cross over
1.	Tendency of genes that are close together on chromosome to be inherited together during inheritance.	Exchange of chromosome segment between non-sister chromatid of homologous chromosome.
2.	It keeps the genes together.	It results in separation of linked genes.
3.	The number of linkage group can never be more than haploid chromosome number.	Frequency of crossing over can never exceed 50%.
4.	It reduce variability.	It increases variability by forming new gene combination.
5.	It provides higher frequency of parental types than recombinant types in test cross progeny.	It provides equal frequency of parental and recombinant types in test cross progeny.
6.	It involve individual chromosome.	It involve non-sister chromatid of homologous chromosome.

INTEXT QUESTIONS

1. Tomato plants having round peach fruits were crossed with having elongated smooth fruits. The F_1 plants were test crossed to yield the following phenotypic classes.

   Round smooth (P_1, RrPp) = 14, Round Peach (P_2, RrPp) = 33

   Elongated smooth (P_3, rrPp) = 141, Elongated Peach (P_4, rrpp) = 12

   Test if the genes for round and peach fruits are linked. If so, in which phase.

2. Plant heterozygous for genes A/a and B/b were selfed to yield the following phenotypic class.

A_B_ = 260, A_bb = 40, aaB_ = 30 aabb = 70

Are the genes A and B linked? If so, in which phase.

....

....

....

....

....

....

....

....

....

....

....

....

....

....

....

....

....

....

....

....

....

....

....

....

Chapter 12

Working Out Problems Related to Gene Mapping

Objectives

- Study of gene mapping.

Introduction

All the genes that are linked together form a linkage group. Genes of a linkage group may be presented on a single straight line in the same order in which they are normally present on the concerned chromosome. The number of different linkage groups in a species is, as a rule, equals to its gametic chromosome number (n). The distance between two neighbouring genes is proportional to the frequency of recombination (%) between them depicted on a line drawing. Such a line drawing depicting the linked genes the recombination frequencies between them is known as Linkage map, Genetic map or Chromosome map. Linkage maps provide information on the genes that are linked together and the frequencies of recombination that may be expected between them. The frequency of recombination between two linked genes cannot exceed 50% which is the frequency in case of independent segregation.

Procedure

For preparing a chromosome map following information are essential.

1. The frequency of recombination between the linked genes.

Recombination frequencies between linked genes are determined from appropriate test crosses. The *per cent* frequencies are used as map units for linkage maps. Recombination of linked genes is accomplished through a process by which homologous chromosome exchange their strictly homologous segments between non-sister chromatids. This process is called Crossing over. (Morgan and Castell, 1912.)

Map unit: A map unit is that distance in a chromosome, which permits one percent recombination (crossing over) between two linked genes. A map unit is also called a centi-Morgan (cM) or Morgan unit.

1% C.O. or 1% Recombination = 1 centi Morgan or 1 Map unit

2. The order or sequence of these genes in the chromosome.
Sequence of linked genes is determined by studying test crosses for three genes at a time (Three point test cross linkage analysis) involving any two of these three genes known and a new gene expected to be linked with them is to be mapped.

Linkage relationship from a three point cross

In a test cross the phenotypes of a progeny is not affected by the test cross parent as it contributes only the recessive alleles of the genes. Three points test cross is expected to produce parental types most frequent and double cross overs the least frequent. The gene order is determined by manipulating the parental combinations into the proper order. Double crossovers usually do not occur between genes less than 5 map units apart. In three point test cross studies, it is desirable to include only those genes that shows < 20%, preferably 10% less, recombination with each other to avoid confusion due to double and triple crossovers.

In maize a test cross for three linked genes e.g. c, sh and wx yields eight types of gametes and phenotypes. The recessiveness of gene "c" responsible for colorlessness "wx" for waxiness and "sh" for shrunken grains. A test cross (CCShShWxWx x ccshshwxwx) yield following progeny.

<table>
<tr><th rowspan="2">Stages of crossing over</th><th colspan="2">F_1 progeny</th><th rowspan="2">Type</th><th rowspan="2">Number</th><th rowspan="2" colspan="2">% Frequency</th></tr>
<tr><th>Genotype</th><th>Phenotype</th></tr>
<tr><td rowspan="2">Non-crossover</td><td>C Sh Wx / c sh wx</td><td>CShWx</td><td>Parental</td><td>2777</td><td>39.7</td><td rowspan="2">78.4</td></tr>
<tr><td>c sh wx / c sh wx</td><td>c sh wx</td><td>Parental</td><td>2708</td><td>38.7</td></tr>
<tr><td rowspan="2">Crossing over (C-Sh)</td><td>C sh wx / c sh wx</td><td>C sh wx</td><td rowspan="2">Single crossover between gene c and sh.</td><td>116</td><td>1.7</td><td rowspan="2">3.5</td></tr>
<tr><td>c sh Wx /c sh wx</td><td>c Sh Wx</td><td>123</td><td>1.8</td></tr>
<tr><td rowspan="2">Crossing over (Sh-Wx)</td><td>C Sh wx / c sh wx</td><td>C Sh wx</td><td rowspan="2">Single crossover between gene sh and wx.</td><td>643</td><td>9.2</td><td rowspan="2">18.1</td></tr>
<tr><td>c sh Wx / c sh wx</td><td>c sh Wx</td><td>626</td><td>8.9</td></tr>
<tr><td rowspan="2">Crossing over (C-Sh) & (Sh-Wx)</td><td>C sh Wx / c sh wx</td><td>C sh Wx</td><td rowspan="2">Double crossover between gene C and sh; Sh and wx</td><td>3</td><td>0.04</td><td rowspan="2">0.1</td></tr>
<tr><td>c Sh wx / c sh wx</td><td>c Sh wx</td><td>4</td><td>0.06</td></tr>
</table>

$$\text{Percent frequency} = \frac{\text{No. of progeny in a phenotypic class}}{\text{Total No. of progeny}} \times 100$$

The double crossover are produced due to simultaneous crossing over between gene C and Sh as well as Sh and Wx. Therefore, the frequencies of double will be added to the estimated recombination frequencies between gene C and Sh and between Sh and Wx, Therefore,

I. Crossing over frequency between genes Sh and Wx will be equal to the sum of frequencies of single crossover types between genes Sh and Wx (18.1) plus the frequencies of double crossover types (0.1%).

   i.e., 18.1 + 0.1 = 18.2% (Y)

II. Crossing over frequency between genes C and Sh will be equals to the sum of frequencies of single crossover types between genes C and Sh (3.5%) plus the frequencies of double cross over types (0.1%).

   i.e., 3.5 + 0.1 = 3.6% (X)

III. Crossing over frequency between genes C and Wx will be equals to the sum of the frequencies of single crossover types between genes C and Sh (3.5%) and the single cross over between genes Sh and Wx (18.1%).

   i.e., 3.5 + 18.1 = 21.6% (Z) excluding double crossovers

   Z = X + Y (21.6 is very close to 3.6 + 18.2)

Therefore, the genes C and Wx must lie on either side of the gene Sh which has to be located between these genes. The real value of Z will be equals to Z+2 × double crossover frequency [21.6 + 2 × 0.1 = 21.8%] (Z = X + Y)

Linkage map: The genes C, Sh and Wx can be mapped in the order C-Sh-Wx at the distance of 3.6 and 18.2 map units, respectively.

C 3.6 Sh 18.2 Wx

Coefficient of coincidence

Double crossovers are produced by two simultaneous crossing over one each on the either side of the gene located between two genes. If the two crossing over are independent of each other, the double crossover could be obtained by multiplying the crossing over percentage of two single crossover between C and Sh (X) and Sh and Wx (Y).

$$\text{Coincidence} = \frac{\text{Observed frequency of double cross overs}}{\text{Expected frequency of double cross overs}}$$

Expected frequency of double crossovers equals to the product of the frequencies of single crossover types between c and sh (X) and wx (Y)

Observed frequency of double cross overs = 0.1%

Expected frequency of double cross overs = 3.6 × 18.2 = 65.52 = 0.66%

Coincidence = 0.66/0.1 = 0.151

The estimated of coefficient of coincidence indicated the degree of agreement between the observed and the expected frequencies of double crossovers.

Coefficient of interference

The occurrence of crossing over in one region of a chromosome interferes with its occurrence in the neighbouring segments called inference. As a rule, the observed frequencies of double crossovers are lower than the expected values. Therefore, the coefficient of interference would be lower when the concerned genes are located close to each other than when they are located farther apart. The intensity of interference may be estimated as coefficient of Interference (C.I).

Coefficient of interference = 1 – coefficient of coincidence

C.I. = 1 – 0.151 = 0.849 or 84.9%.

Example: From the three point test cross mapping experiment, the following genotypic frequencies were obtained.

XyZ	xyz	xYZ	Xyz	XYZ	xyZ	xYz	XYz
2	380	96	109	364	24	3	22

Explain the following

(a) What is the correct gene order?

(b) From the data provided, draw a linkage map showing the distances between the genes.

(c) What is the coefficient of coincidence in this cross?

Solution

(a) For the gene order, we have to compare the double cross over recombinants with parental types. Here changes occur in 'x' gene. So 'x' is in centre and order is YXZ.

(b)

Class	1	2	3	4	5	6	7	8
Genotypes	xyz	XYZ	xYZ	Xyz	xyZ	XYz	XyZ	xYz
Frequency	380	364	96	109	24	22	2	3
Recombinant types	Parental types		Single cross over between 'x' and 'y'.		Single cross over between 'y' and 'z'.		Double cross over types	

Distance between the genes 'x' and 'y' = (class 3 + class 4 + class 7 + class 8)/Total
= 210 / 1000 = 0.21 = 21cM

Distance between the genes 'y' and 'z' = (class 5 + class 6 + class 7 + class 8)/ Total
= 51 / 1000 = 0.051 = 5.1cM

Total = 21 cM + 5.1 cM = 26.1 cM

Linkage map:

Y 21 X 5.1 Z

(c) Coefficient of coincidence(c)= Observed DCO frequency/Expected DCO frequency x100

Observed double cross over frequency = 5/1000 = 0.005

Expected double cross over frequency = 0.21 × 0.051 = 0.01

Therefore, c = 0.005/0.01 = 0.5

Coefficient of interference = 1 – Coefficient of coincidence
= 1 – 0.5 = 0.5

Here, Coefficient of coincidence is 0.5. It indicates the 50% of expected double cross over take place.

INTEXT QUESTIONS

1. Define the following

a. Linkage map

....

....

....

....

....

b. Coefficient of coincidence

....

....

....

....

....

c. Coefficient of interference

....

....

....

....

....

d. Three point test cross

....

....

....

....

....

e. Map unit

....

....

....

....

....

2. A, B, C and D are four genes arranged on same chromosome. If the percentage of recombination between them are-

A – D	10%
A – C	3%
C – D	7%
A – B	5%
C – B	8%

What will be the order of genes on chromosome?

....

....

....

....

....

3. Female Drosophila with cinnabar eye (cn) and vestigial wings (vg) were mated to males with roof wings (rf). The F_1 were all wild-type. When the F_1 females were test crossed with males homozygous for all three traits the following result were obtained.

382	Cinnabar, Vestigial	P
401	Roof	P
3	Cinnabar	DCO1
4	Roof, Vestigial	DCO2
59	Cinnabar, Roof, Vestigial	SCO1
67	Wild	SCO1
44	Cinnabar, Roof	SCO2
40	Vestigial	SCO2

(i) To determine the gene order (rf is not given on the gene map) compare the parental and DCO phenotypes. The correct order of the loci is..............

....

....

....

....

....

(ii) The phenotypes "cinnabar-roof-vestigial" and "wild" were formed as a result of a single crossover between .... and ....

Calculated map distance.

....

....

....

....

....

....

Chapter 13

Working Out Problems Related to Multiple Alleles

Objectives

- Better understand the phenomenon of multiple alleles.

Introduction

The word allele is a general term to denote the alternative forms of a gene or contrasting gene pair that denote the alternative form of a gene is called allele. These alleles were previously considered by Bateson as hypothetical partner in Mendelian segregation. Mendel and his followers used the term 'allele' or 'alleleomorph' to denote the alternative form of the normal gene. It means the genes for tall and dwarf characters of pea plant are alleles. The former is normal or wild allele and the later is mutant allele. A gene can mutate several times producing several alternative expressions. When three or more alleles are found for any particular gene, these are called 'multiple alleles'. These occupy the same locus in homologous chromosomes.

Multiple alleles are defined as genes that are members of the same gene pair and are located on the same locus. All of them control the same character but each of the allele affects that character somewhat differently than the others. In any diploid organism, a particular gene pair is represented by two alleles of the series, one allele on each of the two chromosomes of a homologous pair. This is because an organism has just two chromosomes of each type. These form a homologous pair. However, in the individuals of a population or species, many alternative forms of the same gene may be present. The grouping of all the possible alleles of a gene pair is defined as a system of multiple alleles and their mode of inheritance is called multiple allelism. The multiple allele system can be represented as A1, A2, A3, A4 etc.

Characters of Multiple Alleles

- The study of multiple alleles may be done in population.
- Multiple alleles occupy the same locus within the homologous chromosomes. It means only one member of the series is present in a given chromosome.

- Since only two chromosomes of each type are present in each diploid cell, only two genes of the multiple series are found in a cell and also in a given individual.
- The gametes contain only one chromosome of each type, therefore, only one allele of the multiple series in each gamete.
- There is no crossing over between the members of multiple alleles. Crossing over takes place between two different genes only (inter-generic recombination) and does not occur within a gene (intragenic recombination).
- Multiple alleles control the same character, but each of them is characterised by different manifestations. Sturtevant has summarised it as "they carry the same function but with varying degree of efficiency".
- The multiple alleles of a series are more often related as dominant and recessive. More commonly, the normal gene is dominant to all other mutant alleles. Even the intermediate members of the series may be related as dominant and recessive, or they may exhibit co-dominance.
- Multiple alleles never show complementation with each other. By complementation test the allelic and non-allelic genes may be differentiated well. The production of wild type phenotype in a trans-heterozygote for 2 mutant alleles is known as complementation test.
- Multiple alleles have been studied in Rabbits, Guinea pigs, Mice, Drosophila and Man.

Examples of multiple alleles

Blood group in human : 3 alleles
Coat colour in rabbit : 4 alleles
Self-incompatibility in plant: : 3 alleles
Eye colour in drosophila : 15 alleles

If 'n' is the number of alleles of a gene then number of different possible genotypes is –

Possible genotypes = n (n +1)/2

Blood Groups in Human

It was found that all persons could be classified in to four groups with regard to the antigen property of the blood cells. Large number of persons have been classified in to these four groups by means of the agglutination test and the distribution of blood groups in the offspring of parents of known blood groups has been studied. The evidence shows that these blood properties are determined by a series of three allelic genes I^A, I^B and i, as follows:

I^A : Dominant I^B : Dominant i : Recessive

I^A is a gene for the production of the antigen A. I^B for antigen B, and i for neither antigen. The existence of these alleles in man and the case with which the blood groups can be identified have obvious practical applications in blood transfusion, cases of disputed percentage and description of human populations.

The alleles of these genes which affect a variety of biochemical properties of the blood, act in such a way that in the heterozygous compound I^AI^B, each allele exhibits its own characteristics and specific effect. The cells of the heterozygote contain both antigens A and B. On the other hand, I^A and I^B both show complete dominance over i, which lacks both antigens.

Table 1. Systematic information about antigen and antibodies of different blood groups and their transfusions.

Blood group	**Genotypes**	**Antigen on RBC**	**Antibody**	**Safe Transfusions**	
				From	**To**
AB	I^AI^B	A, B	None	A, B, AB, O	AB
B	I^BI^B or I^Bi	B	a	B, O	B, AB
A	I^AI^A or I^Ai	A	b	A, O	A, AB
O	ii	None	a, b	O	A, B, AB, O
I^A: Dominant I^B: Dominant i : Recessive					

Table 2. Showing phenotype results from different blood groups

Genotype	**AA or AO**	**BB or BO**	**AB**	**OO**
Phenotype	Type A Carbohydrate	Type B Carbohydrate	Type A and B Carbohydrate	No Carbohydrate
Blood Group	Group A 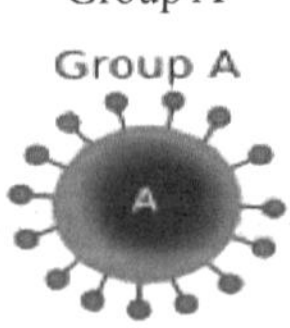	Group B 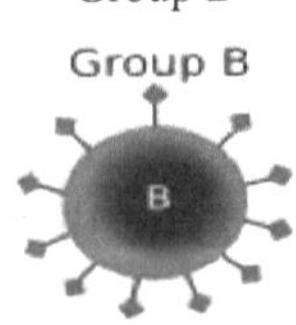	Group AB 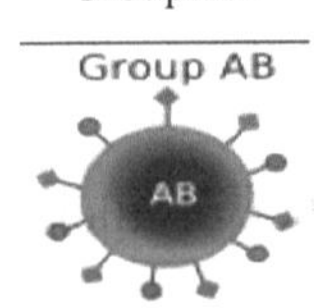	Group OO 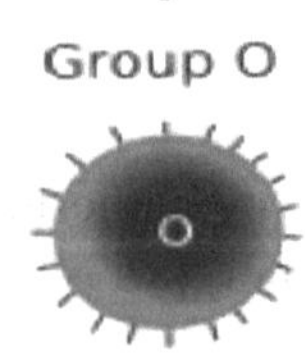

Table 3. Showing possible blood types of children from parents of various blood groups in O x AB line column 3 instead of A.B write A, B

Parents		**Children**	
Phenotypes	**Genotypes**	**Phenotypes**	**Genotypes**
O × O	ii × ii	O	ii
O × A	ii × I^AI^A or I^Ai	O, A	ii, I^Ai
O × B	ii × I^BI^B or I^Bi	O, B	ii, I^Bi
O × AB	ii × I^AI^B	A, B	I^Ai, I^Bi
A × A	I^AI^A or I^Ai × I^AI^A or I^Ai	A, O	I^AI^A, ii

Parents		Children	
Phenotypes	**Genotypes**	**Phenotypes**	**Genotypes**
A × B	I^AI^A or I^Ai × I^BI^B or I^Bi	A, AB, O, B	I^Ai, I^AI^B, ii, I^Bi
A × AB	I^AI^A or I^Ai × I^AI^B	A, B, AB	I^AI^A, I^Bi, I^AI^B
B × B	I^BI^B or I^Bi × I^BI^B or I^Bi	B, O	I^BI^B, ii
B × AB	I^BI^B or I^Bi × I^AI^B	A, B, AB	I^AI^A, I^BI^B, I^AI^B
AB × AB	I^AI^B × I^AI^B	A, B, AB	I^AI^A, I^BI^B, I^AI^B

Coat Colour in Rabbit

The colour of the skin in rabbits is influenced by a series of multiple alleles. There are four alleles for coat colour in rabbit. The normal colour of the skin is brown. Besides it there are white races called albino and Himalayan as the mutant races. The Himalayan is similar to albino but has darker nose, ear, feet and tail. The mutant genes albino (a) and Himalayan (ah) occupy the same locus and are allelic. Both albino and Himalayan are recessive to their normal allele (+).

Table 4. Characteristics of coat colour in rabbit and their possible genotypes.

Phenotype	Symbol	Possible genotypes	Characteristics
Agouti	A	AA, Aa^{ch}, Aa^h, Aa	Wild type, full coloured.
Chinchila	a^{ch}	$a^{ch}a^{ch}$, $a^{ch}a^h$, $a^{ch}a$	Mixed colours and white hairs.
Himalayan	a^h	a^ha^h, a^ha	White with black tip on extremities like nose, tail and feet.
Albino	a	aa	Colourless (white races).

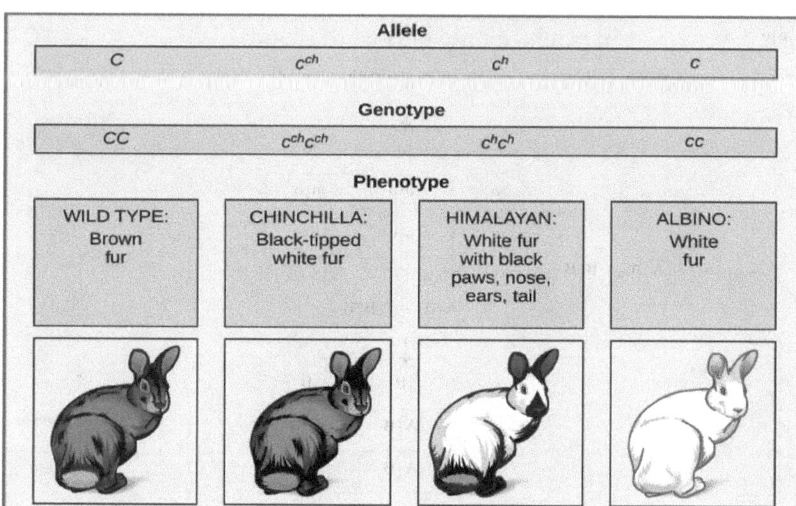

Fig. Coat colour in rabbit

These alleles show a gradient in dominance: $A > a^{ch} > a^h > a$

A cross between an albino and Himalayan produces a Himalayan in the F_1 and not intermediate as is usual in the case of other multiple alleles.

	Albino	×	Himalayan		
	a/a	↓	a^h/a^h		
F_1		a^h/a (Himalayan)			
	a^h/a	×	a^h/a	(Selfing)	
F_2	a^h/a^h :	a^h/a	: a^h/a	:	a/a
		3	:		1
		Himalayan	:		Albino

(Representing a cross between an Albino and Himalayan races of rabbits)

Problem: In humans, there are four types of blood; type A, type B, type AB, and type O. The alleles A and B are codominant to each other and the O allele is recessive to both A and B alleles. So a person with the genotype AA or AO will have A type of blood.

(a) What possible genotypes will produce B type of blood? _____________

(b) What is the only genotype that will produce O type of blood? ___________

(c) What is the only genotype that will produce AB type of blood? ________

Solution:

(a) Possible genotypes that produces B type blood group – I^BI^B and I^BI^O

(b) I^oI^o genotype will produce only O type of blood.

$$I^oI^o \text{ x } I^oI^o$$
$$\downarrow$$

	I^o	I^o
I^o	I^oI^o	I^oI^o
I^o	I^oI^o	I^oI^o

(c) Genotype I^AI^A x I^BI^B will produce only AB type of blood

$$I^AI^A \text{ x } I^BI^B$$
$$\downarrow$$

	I^B	I^B
I^A	I^AI^B	I^AI^B
I^A	I^AI^B	I^AI^B

Problem: You are blood type O and you marry a person with blood type AB. Complete a Punnett square for this cross. List the possible blood types (phenotypes) of your offspring.

Solution: When a parent with O blood group marry with AB blood group, then Punnet square for this cross formed as

I^OI^O x I^AI^B

↓

	I^A	I^B
I^o	I^AI^O	I^BI^O
I^o	I^AI^O	I^BI^O

Result: Phenotype of offsprings are A type and B type blood group.

INTEXT QUESTIONS

1. Define Multiple allele with suitable examples.

....

....

....

....

....

2. What will be the possible number of genotypes in case of coat colour in rabbit and ABO blood group in human?

....

....

....

....

....

3. A homologous agouti rabbit crossed with albino rabbit. What is the percentage of impure agouti in F_2 generation?

....

....

....

....

....

4. A man of 'A' blood group marries with a women of 'AB' blood group. Which type of progeny would indicate the men is heterozygous 'A'.

   i. AB ii. A iii. O iv. B

....

....

....

....

....

5. If one parent has a blood group 'A' and the other parent has blood group 'B'. The offspring's have which blood group.

i. AB ii. O iii. BO iv. A, B, AB, O

....

....

....

....

....

6. A child blood group is 'O'. His parent's blood group cannot be -

i. B, O ii. A, O iii. AB iv. A, B

....

....

....

....

....

Chapter 14

Study of Different Types of Gene Interactions and Modification of the Typical Dihybrid F_2 Ratios

Objectives

- Better understand the various types of gene interaction.

Introduction

Gene interaction is the phenomenon of two or more genes that affect each other's expression in different ways in the development of a single character of an organism. It is the modification of normal phenotypic expression of gene due to interaction between alleles or non-alleles. In such situation, two or more than two genes may interact to give rise to a particular phenotype.

The following observations and assumptions are found in gene interactions:

1. Genes that interact with each other are present on different loci and unlinked, assort separately during gamete formation.
2. If complete dominance exists between the alleles of any gene pair or both the gene pairs, such as AA and Aa or BB and Bb, then the same genetic effects are observed.
3. All P_1 crosses will involve homozygous individuals i.e., AABB × aabb or AAbb × aaBB. Therefore, F_1 generation always has only heterozygous genotype i.e., AaBb.
4. The results of F_2 generation are conclusive. With two pairs of genes F_2 genotypic ratio is 9:3:3:1= 16 i.e., AABB = 9/16, AAbb = 3/16, aaBB = 3/16 and aabb = 1/16. In gene interaction, this F_2 ratio is variously modified.

Two types of interaction

A. Allelic interaction

This interaction takes place between the alleles of a gene, controlling a single character, which are present on homologous chromosome. This interaction involves one gene pair. It is also called as inter-allelic or intra-genic interaction. Example: Dominance, co-dominance, incomplete dominance.

B. Non-allelic interaction

This interaction takes place between the different pairs alleles of genes, influencing a character, which are present on non-homologous chromosome. This interaction involves two gene pair. It is also called as inter-genic interaction.

Examples of non-allelic interaction –

1. Epistasis:

The term epistasis was coined by Bateson in 1909. Epistasis (act of stopping) is the interaction between non-allelic genes in which one gene pair masks, inhibits or suppresses the expression of other gene pair, which is located on non-homologous chromosome. The gene that suppresses the expression of other gene is known as inhibiting or epistatic gene and the gene whose effect is masked is known as hypostatic gene. Epistasis leads to modification of normal dihybrid or trihybrid segregation ratio in F_2 generation.

Epistasis can be mainly of two types:

1. a. **Dominant epistasis**

In this case, epistatic gene suppress the expression of another non-allelic gene, when it is present in dominant form.

E.g. Fruit colour in *cucurbita pepo* - Two gene pair [(A, a) and (B, b)] control fruit colour.

B : Yellow	**9** A_B_ : White	
b : Green	**3** A_bb : White	
A* : White	**3** aaB_ : Yellow	
(*Epistatic gene)	**1** aabb : Green	
Modified Phenotype -	**12** White: **3** Yellow : **1** Green	**12:3:1**
Test cross ratio -	**2** White: **1** Yellow: **1** Green	**2:1:1**

2. b. **Recessive epistasis**

In this case, epistatic gene suppress the expression of another non-allelic gene, when it is present in homozygous recessive condition.

Example:

Bulb colour in onion. Two gene pair [(A, a) and (B, b)] control bulb colour.

B : Red	**9** A_B_ : Red	
b : Yellow	**3** A_bb : Yellow	
a* : White	**3** aaB_ : White	
(*Epistatic gene)	**1** aabb : White	
Modified Phenotype -	**9** White: **3** Yellow: **4** Green	**9:3:4**
Test cross ratio -	**1** White: **1** Yellow: **2** Green	**1:1:2**

2. Inhibitory gene action

In this type of interaction, a dominant allele at one locus can mask the expression of both (dominant and recessive) alleles at second locus. This is also known as inhibitory gene interaction. Inhibitory gene supress the expression of dominant non-allelic gene when it is present in dominant form. Inhibitory gene does not produce its own phenotype. In this case, suppressed gene behave as a recessive gene.

E.g. Leaf colour in rice.

B : Purple		**9** A_B_ : Green
b : Green		**3** A_bb : Green
A* : Inhibitory gene		**3** aaB_ : Purple
		1 aabb : Green
Modified Phenotype -	**13** Green : **3** Purple	**13:3**
Test cross ratio -	**1** Purple: **3** Green	**1:3**

3. Duplicate gene effect / Duplicate dominant epistasis

When a dominant allele at either of two loci can mask the expression of recessive alleles at the two loci, it is known as duplicate dominant epistasis.

In this interaction, when two non-allelic gene separately present in dominant form they produce same phenotype. If they are present together in dominant form they also produce same phenotype. In this condition, both the non-allelic genes are duplicate to each other for the production of a particular phenotype.

In this interaction, only one dominant gene of any gene pair is sufficient to produce a particular phenotype.

E.g.

i. Floating habit in rice – Floating, non-floating
ii. Fruit shape in *Capsella* – G.H. Shull observed this interaction on Shepherd's purse plant belonging to genus *Capsella*.

Two kind of phenotype with respect to fruit shape were known – Triangular capsule and Top shaped capsule.

	9 A_B_ : Triangular capsule	
	3 A_bb : Triangular capsule	
	3 aaB_ : Triangular capsule	
	1 aabb : Top shaped capsule	
Modified Phenotype -	**15** Triangular : **1** Top shaped	**15:1**
Test cross ratio -	**3** Triangular: **1** Top shaped	**3:1**

4. Additive gene action/Polymeric gene action/Duplicate recessive epistasis

In this case, two genes controlling a character produces identical phenotype when they are alone *i.e.* with the homozygous recessive condition of the other gene. But when both the genes are present together, their phenotype effect is enhanced as if the effect of the two genes were cumulative or additives. It should be noted that in this case both the genes show complete dominance.

E.g. Fruit shape in *cucurbita pepo*

9 A_B_	:	Discoid
3 A_bb	:	Spherical
3 aaB_	:	Spherical
1 aabb	:	Cylindrical

Modified Phenotype -	**9** Discoid : **6** Spherical : **1** Cylindrical	**9:6:1**
Test cross ratio -	**1** Discoid : **2** Spherical : **1** Cylindrical	**1:2:1**

5. Collaborative gene action / Modified gene action/Typical dihybrid ratio

In this interaction, two dominant non-allelic gene produce different phenotype when separately present. If they present together in dominant form they produce totally new phenotype due to their collaboration.

E.g. Comb shape in fowl (Poultry)

9 A_B_	:	Walnut
3 A_bb	:	Rose
3 aaB_	:	Pea
1 aabb	:	Single

Modified Phenotype -	**9** Walnut : **3** Rose : **3** Pea : **1** Single	**9:3:3:1**
Test cross ratio -	**1** Walnut : **1** Rose : **1** Pea : **1** Single	**1:1:1:1**

6. Complementary gene action

When recessive alleles at either of the two loci can mask the expression of dominant the two loci, it is called duplicate recessive epistasis. In this interaction, two non-allelic genes are essential in dominant form to produce a specific phenotype. If any one of the genes or both the gene pair present in total recessive condition then particular phenotype is not expressed.

E.g. Flower colour in *Lathyrus odoratus* (Sweet pea)

9 A_B_	:	Purple
3 A_bb	:	White
3 aaB_	:	White
1 aabb	:	White

Modified Phenotype -	**9** Purple : **7** White	**9:7**
Test cross ratio -	**1** Purple : **3** White	**1:3**

7. Supplementary gene action

Here one dominant gene has its own phenotypic effect and other dominant gene has no effect of its own but its presence with the first gene modified the phenotypic expression. Thus in supplementary gene action the dominant allele of one gene is necessary for the development of the concerned phenotype, while the other gene modifies the expression of the first gene.

E.g. Coat colour in mice

B :	Balck	**9** A_B_	: Agouti
b :	Albino	**3** A_bb	: Albino
A* :	*Supplementary gene	**3** aaB_	: Black
		1 aabb	: Albino
Modified Phenotype -	**9** Agouti: **3** Black: **4** Albino	**9:3:4**	
Test cross ratio -	**1** Agouti: **1** Black: **2** Albino	**1:1:2**	

Problem: In poultry rose comb and pea comb patterns are produced by the dominant effect of two different genes. The recessive nature of both these alleles generates a single comb. But a new type known as walnut was also produced along with rose, pea, and single in 9:3:3:1 ratio in a cross between rose combed and pea combed fowls. Suggest the possible of F_1 and F_2 offspring genotypes and explain the type of gene interaction involved in this cross.

Explanation

1. R gene in homozygous or heterozygous state and in the absence of 'P' produces Rose comb in fowls.
2. P gene in homozygous or heterozygous state and in the absence of' R' produces Pea comb.
3. When both R & P comes together they interact and produces a novel character Walnut in F_1 generation.
4. Both the recessive genes interact and produces single comb.
5. Even though the F_2 ratio is numerically same as a dihybrid ratio it is not at all related to the pattern of inheritance. Because the F_1 is a different

character not seen among the parents. The F_2 single is also not seen anywhere in the parental lines. The cross can be shown as follows.

Phenotype of parents: Rose × Pea

Genotype of parents: RRpp × rrPP

↓

F_1 Offspring - RrPp (Walnut)

↓ Selfing

RrPp × RrPp

↓

	RP	Rp	rP	rp
RP	RRPP	RRPp	RrPP	RrPp
Rp	RRPp	RRpp	RrPp	Rrpp
rP	RrPP	RrPp	rrPP	rrPp
rp	RrPp	Rrpp	rrPp	rrpp

The F_2 ratio – 9 walnut : 3rose: 3pea: 1single

Problem: Two white flowered strains of sweet peas were crossed, producing an F_1 with only purple flowers. Random crossing among the F_1 produced 96 progeny plants of which 53 are purple, 43 with white flowers.

(a) What phenotypic ratio is shown by the F_2?

(b) What type of interaction is involved?

(c) What were the probable genotypes of the parental strains?

Explanation

Firstly find out the possible ratio and find out the type of interaction.

Total number of offspring = 96.

Find out the proportion of the first group of offspring among the sum total of 560. We are considering it, as a multiple of 16. (Dihybrid cross)

So the first group is- 53 × 16 / 96 = 8.83 = 9 purple

The second group is – 43 × 16 / 96 = 7.16 = 7 white

It is a case of complementary factor interaction. Here we will get a ratio of 9:7. Explain the theory of complementary factor interaction. The genotype of parental strains – ccPp (white) × Ccpp (white). C -- in single dose or double dose produce white flower colour. Likewise P-- in single dose or double dose produce white flower colour. But when they come together they interact and produce purple flower colour. The double recessives will also produce white. The last three groups of Mendelian ratio of 9:3:3:1 is indistinguishable and modified to 9:7 ratio.

Problem: Crosses were made between two types of Oats. One with white hulled and the other with black hulled and the F_2 had 178 black, 126 grey and 26 white. Give the type of interaction and explain it.

Answer:

Firstly find out the possible ratio and find out the type of interaction.
Total number of offspring = 178 + 126 + 26 = 330
Find out the proportion of the first group of offspring among the sum total of 330. We are considering it, as a multiple of 16. (Dihybrid cross)
So the first group is –178 × 16/330 = 8.63 = 9 black
The second group is –126 × 16/330 = 6.01 = 6 grey.
The third group is –26 × 16/330 = 1.26 = 1 white.

Explanation

It is a case of dominant and recessive interaction. There are two pairs of genes, which produces the same character separately. When they come together they interact and produce a novel character. When both the recessive genes come they interact and produce another character. For example if the genes are R-- & B-- interact and produce black colour. The genes R alone produce grey and gene B alone produces grey. Both the recessive genes interact and produce white. In the Mendelian ratio 9:3:3:1, the two middle groups are indistinguishable and so modified to 9:6:1. The F_1 are all black and F_2 are segregated to - 9 black: 6 grey: 1 white.

Summary

S. No.	Gene interaction	Modified phenotypic ratio	Modified testcross ratio	Examples
1.	Dominant epistasis	12:3:1	2:1:1	Fruit colour in *cucurbita pepo*
2.	Recessive epistasis	9:3:4	1:1:2	Bulb colour in onion
3.	Inhibitory gene action	13:3	1:3	Leaf colour in rice

S. No.	Gene interaction	Modified phenotypic ratio	Modified testcross ratio	Examples
4.	Duplicate gene action/ Duplicate dominant epistasis	15:1	3:1	Floating habit in rice, Fruit shape in *Capsella*
5.	Additive gene action / Polymeric gene action / Duplicate recessive epistasis	9:6:1	1:2:1	Fruit shape in ***cucurbita pepo***
6.	Collaborative gene action/ Modified gene action/ Typical dihybrid ratio	9:3:3:1	1:1:1:1	Comb shape in fowl (Poultry)
7.	Complementary gene action	9:7	1:3	Flower colour in *Lathyrus odoratus* (Sweet pea)
8.	Supplementary gene action	9:3:4	1:1:2	Coat colour in mice

INTEXT QUESTIONS

1. Define the following.

(i) Epistasis

....

....

....

....

....

(ii) Complementary gene action

....

....

....

....

....

(iii) Duplicate gene action

....

....

....

....

....

2. Four walnut hens are crossed to single and each produces a large number of chicks. The first produces only walnuts, the second produces only walnuts and peas, the third produces only walnuts and rose and the fourth produces among other types single also. Give the genotypes of each of the four walnut hens used as parents..

....

....

....

....

....

3. In summer squash spherical fruit is recessive to disc. Spherical races from different geographical regions were crossed. The F_1 were disc and the F_2 were segregated to 35 discs, 25 spherical, 4 elongate. Explain the result?

....

....

....

....

....

Chapter 15

Working Out Problems Related to Probability

Objectives

- Better understand the phenomenon of probability.

Introduction

The concept of probability is basis to many principles of classical genetics (segregation, independent assortment etc.) The principals of population genetics are based on the considerations of laws of probability. Probability is the likelihood of occurrence of an event.

Trial

A trial refers to an opportunity provided for an event to occur, e.g. tossing of a coin once constitute one trial as it provides an opportunity for head or tail to occur. A new borne can be either a boy or a girl.

Event

An event is the occurrence of something. The occurrence of head or tail in a toss is an event. A new born baby boy or girl is also an event. The events that occur purely due to chance are grouped into two categories on the basis of their relationship with each other (i) Mutually exclusive events (ii) Independent events.

Important concepts of probability

Basic formula of probability

$$\text{Probability of an event (P)} = \frac{\text{Number of times in which the event occurs}}{\text{Total number of trials}}$$

Problem: What is the probability of rolling a 5 when a die is rolled?

Solution: On rolling die, number of time a 5 occur = 1
Total number of possible outcome = 6
Probability of rolling a 5 when a die is rolled = 1/6

Compound probability

It is defined as the likelihood of occurrence of more than one outcome.

Formula of compound probability

$$P(A \text{ or } B) = P(A) + P(B) - P(A \text{ and } B)$$

Where, A and B are any two events.

P(A or B) – Probability of occurrence of atleast one of the events.

P(A and B) – Probability of occurrence of A and B at the same time.

Mutually exclusive events

Such events are so related among themselves that the occurrence of one of them in a trial prevents the occurrence of the remaining events in the same trial. Thus in trial, the occurrence of head excluded that of tail and the occurrence of boy excludes that of girl and vice- versa. In other words, we can say "the occurrence of one event indicate the non-occurrence of another events." For mutually exclusive events P(A and B) = 0.

Problem: What is the probability of getting a 2 or a 5 when a die is rolled?

Solution: Taking the individual probabilities of each number, getting a 2 is 1/6 and so is getting a 5.

Applying the formula of compound probability,

Probability of getting a 2 or a 5,

$$\begin{aligned} P(2 \text{ or } 5) &= P(2) + P(5) - P(2 \text{ and } 5) \\ &= 1/6 + 1/6 - 0 \\ &= 2/6 = 1/3. \end{aligned}$$

Problem: Consider the example of finding the probability of selecting a black card or a 6 from a deck of 52 cards.

Solution: We need to find out P(B or 6)

Probability of selecting a black card = 26/52

Probability of selecting a 6 = 4/52

Probability of selecting both a black card and a 6 = 2/52

$$\begin{aligned} P(B \text{ or } 6) &= P(B) + P(6) - P(B \text{ and } 6) \\ &= 26/52 + 4/52 - 2/52 \\ &= 28/52 \\ &= 7/13 \end{aligned}$$

Independent events

When two or more events are so related that the occurrence of one of the events does not affect the probability of the remaining events, they are referred to as independent events. When two coins, A and B, are tossed together or separately, the occurrence of head or tail in case of I^{st} coin (A) does not affect the probability of occurrence of head or tail in the II_{nd} coin (B). Hence the occurrence of head or tail in coin A is independent of that in coin B. Therefore, they are known as independent events.

The probability of occurrence of two or more independent events together is the product of individual probabilities of these events.

Problem: Say, a coin is tossed twice. What is the probability of getting two consecutive tails?

Solution Probability of getting a tail in one toss = 1/2

The coin is tossed twice. So 1/2 * 1/2 = 1/4 is the answer.

Here's the verification of the above answer with the help of sample space.

When a coin is tossed twice, the sample space is {(H,H), (H,T), (T,H), (T,T)}.

Our desired event is (T,T) whose occurrence is only once out of four possible outcomes and hence, our answer is 1/4.

Problem: Consider another example where a pack contains 4 blue, 2 red and 3 black pens. If a pen is drawn at random from the pack, replaced and the process repeated 2 more times. What is the probability of drawing 2 blue pens and 1 black pen?

Solution:

Here, total number of pens = 9
Probability of drawing 1 blue pen = 4/9
Probability of drawing another blue pen = 4/9
Probability of drawing 1 black pen = 3/9
Probability of drawing 2 blue pens and 1 black pen = 4/9 * 4/9 * 3/9
= 48/729 = 16/243

Table 1. Probability of different combinations of head (H) and tail (T) obtained on tossing of two coins (A and B) simultaneously or separate.

S. No.	Coin A	Coin B	Probability	Class (2n) = 4
1.	H	H	1/2/ × 1/2 = 1/4	H in both coins
2.	H	T	1/2/ × 1/2 = 1/4	H in A and T in B
3.	T	H	1/2/ × 1/2 = 1/4	T in A and H in B
4	T	T	1/2/ × 1/2 = 1/4	T in both coins

The probability of getting one 'H' and one 'T' on tossing of two coins once will be the sum of the probabilities of these two combination = (1/4 + 1/4 = 1/2) because such combination of independent events behaves as mutually exclusive events.

Table 2. Probability of different combination of H and T obtained after tossing of three coins (A, B and C).

S. No.	Coin A	Coin B	Coin C	Probability	Class 2n = 8	
1.	H	H	H	1/2 × 1/2 ×1/2 = 1/8	HHH = 3H	1/8
2.	H	H	T	1/2 × 1/2 × 1/2 = 1/8	HHT = 2 H 1T	
3.	H	T	H	1/2 × 1/2 ×1/2 = 1/8	HTH= 2 2H 1T	3/8
4.	T	H	H	1/2 × 1/2 × 1/2 = 1/8	THH = 2H 1T	
5.	H	T	T	1/2 × 1/2 × 1/2 = 1/8	HTT = 2 T 1H	
6.	T	H	T	1/2 × 1/2 × 1/2 = 1/8	HTT = 2T 1H	3/8
7.	T	T	H	1/2 × 1/2 × 1/2 = 1/8	TTH = 2T 1H	
8.	T	T	T	1/2 × 1/2 × 1/2 = 1/8	TTT = 3T	1/8

Dependent Events

When two events occur, if the outcome of one event affects the outcome of the other, they are referred to as dependent events.

Problem: A pack contains 4 blue, 2 red and 3 black pens. If 2 pens are drawn at random from the pack, NOT replaced and then another pen is drawn. What is the probability of drawing 2 blue pens and 1 black pen?

Solution:

Probability of drawing 1 blue pen = 4/9
Probability of drawing another blue pen = 3/8
Probability of drawing 1 black pen = 3/7
Probability of drawing 2 blue pens and 1 black pen = 4/9 * 3/8 * 3/7 = 1/14

Problem: What is the probability of drawing a king and a queen consecutively from a deck of 52 cards, without replacement?

Solution:
Probability of drawing a king = 4/52 = 1/13
After drawing one card, the number of cards are 51.
Probability of drawing a queen = 4/51.
Now, the probability of drawing a king and queen consecutively is 1/13 * 4/51 = 4/663

Conditional probability

Conditional probability is calculating the probability of an event given that another event has already occurred.

The formula for conditional probability P(A|B), read as P(A given B) is

$$P(A|B) = P\ (A \text{ and } B)\ /\ P(B)$$

Problem: In a class, 40% of the students study math and science. 60% of the students study math. What is the probability of a student studying science given he/she is already studying math?

Solution:
P(M and S) = 0.40
P(M) = 0.60
P(S|M) = P(M and S)/P(M) = 0.40/0.60 = 2/3 = 0.67

Complement of an event

A complement of an event A can be stated as that which does NOT contain the occurrence of A. A complement of an event is denoted as P(Ac) or P(A').

$$P(Ac) = 1 - P(A)$$

or it can be stated, P(A) + P(Ac) = 1

For example:

- If A is the event of getting a head in coin toss, Ac is not getting a head i.e., getting a tail.
- If A is the event of getting an even number in a die roll, Ac is the event of NOT getting an even number i.e., getting an odd number.
- If A is the event of randomly choosing a number in the range of –3 to 3, Ac is the event of choosing every number that is NOT negative i.e., 0,1,2 & 3 (0 is neither positive or negative).

Problem: A single coin is tossed 5 times. What is the probability of getting at least one head?

Solution: Consider solving this using complement.

Probability of getting no head = P(all tails) = 1/32

P(at least one head) = 1 – P(all tails) = 1 – 1/32 = 31/32.

INTEXT QUESTIONS

1. What is the probability of the drawing an ace from a pack of cards?

....

....

....

....

....

2. What is the probability of the drawing either an ace or a queen from a pack of cards?

....

....

....

....

....

3. What is the probability of getting -
   (a) A 5 with a single dice.

....

....

....

....

....

   (b) A 5 each of two dice thrown simultaneously.

....

....

....

....

....

(c) Any combination totalling 7 on two dice thrown simultaneously?

....

....

....

....

....

NOTE SHEET

References

Rangaswamy, R. 2016. A Textbook of Agricultural Statistics, New Age International Publishers.

Singh, B. D. 2014. Fundamental of Genetics, Kalyani Publishers

Singh, P. 2016. Elements of Genetics, Kalyani Publishers

Strickberger, M. W. 1968. Genetics. 1968. MacMillan, New York.

http://vlab.amrita.edu/?sub=3&brch=188&sim=1102&cnt=2

http://www.biologydiscussion.com/chromosomes/study-notes-on-chromosome-technique/39301

http://www.biologydiscussion.com/genetics/multiple-alleles/multiple-alleles-meaning-characteristics-and-examples-genes/35452

http://www.funscience.in/study-zone/Physics/OpticalInstruments/CompoundMicroscope.php #sthash.iCTQrbBT.dpbs

http://www.yourarticlelibrary.com/micro-biology/working-principle-and-parts-of-a-simple-microscope-with-diagrams/26490

http://www.yourarticlelibrary.com/micro-biology/working-principle-and-parts-of-a-compound-microscope-with-diagrams/26509

https://people.smp.uq.edu.au/YoniNazarathy/stat_models_B_course_spring_07/distributions/chisqtab.pdf

https://microbenotes.com/simple-microscope-principle-instrumentation-and-applications/

FSC
www.fsc.org
MIX
Papier | Fördert
gute Waldnutzung
FSC® C083411

Zeitfracht Medien GmbH
Ferdinand-Jühlke-Straße 7
99095 Erfurt, Deutschland
produktsicherheit@kolibri360.de